Urticaria and Angioedema

Torsten Zuberbier • Clive Grattan • Marcus Maurer

Urticaria and Angioedema

Springer

Prof. Dr. med. Torsten Zuberbier
Department of Dermatology and Allergy
Allergy-centre-Charité
Charité-Universitätsmedizin Berlin
Charitéplatz 1
10117 Berlin
Germany
Email: torsten.zuberbier@charite.de

Prof. Dr. med. Marcus Maurer
Department of Dermatology and Allergy
Allergy-centre-Charité
Charité-Universitätsmedizin Berlin
Charitéplatz 1
10117 Berlin
Germany
Email: marcus.maurer@charite.de

Clive E. H. Grattan, MA, MD, FRCP
Department of Dermatology
Norfolk and Norwich University Hospital
Norwich
NR4 7UY
United Kingdom
Email: clive.grattan@nnuh.nhs.uk

ISBN: 978-3-540-79047-1 e-ISBN: 978-3-540-79048-8

DOI: 10.1007/978-3-540-79048-8

Springer Heidelberg Dordrecht London New York

Library of Congress Control Number: 2009934505

Cover design: eStudioCalamar, Figueres/Berlin

Printed on acid-free paper

Springer is part of Springer Science+Business Media (www.springer.com)

Preface

Urticaria is one of the most common diseases in dermatology and allergy. Unlike many other diseases, the fleeting nature of the wheals makes first diagnosis by both patients and physicians in many cases easy. However, this only refers to the ordinary wheals. The disease itself is highly complex in nature, with variety of clinical manifestations ranging from pinpoint-sized wheals to extensive angiodema. Complexity is also seen in the diversity of possible eliciting factors, the many different clinical subtypes and the therapeutic responsiveness.

Only in recent years has a better understanding of the diversity in the different subtypes led to new classifications and new evidence-based guidelines for diagnostics and management of the disease. While mast cells are in the center of most urticaria reactions, it is now clearly understood that the responsible mediators are not only limited to histamines.

The current book appears in a series of books by Springer. In 1986, the first monograph was edited by Professor Henz née Chanewsky. Since then, two updates of the book have appeared in the German language with Professor Henz as first editor and T. Zuberbier, J. Grabbe, and E. Monroe as the co-editors of the most recent English version, published in 1998. All these books have been written as a joint effort of Professor Henz together with her team at the Department of Dermatology at the Virchow Clinic, Humboldt University, Berlin.

With the retirement of Professor Henz from her chair as head of the department of dermatology and novel guidelines available, the current group of editors has taken up the task of developing a completely new setup for the book. A group of internationally known authors in the field of urticaria have been asked to write different chapters, focusing on practical guidelines regarding diagnosis and therapy.

This book is designed to be a useful reference for dermatologists, allergologists, pediatricians, and practitioners in general medicine, laying out clear-cut standard operating procedures on how to manage this disease efficiently.

Berlin, Germany — Prof. Dr. Torsten Zuberbier
Norwich, UK — Dr. Clive Grattan
Berlin, Germany — Prof. Dr. Marcus Maurer

Contents

Contributors

Ilaria Baiardini
Allergy and Respiratory Diseases,
Department of Internal Medicine,
Genoa University, Genoa, Italy
ilaria.baiardini@libero.it

Carsten Bindslev-Jensen, MD, PhD, DMSci
Department of Dermatology and Allergy
Centre, Odense University Hospital
and University of Southern Denmark,
5000 Odense, Denmark
carsten.bindslev-jensen@ouh.regionsyd-danmark.dk

Elena Borzova
Department of Dermatology, Norfolk and
Norwich University Hospital,
Norwich NR4 7UY, UK
elena.borzova@nnuh.nhs.uk

Fulvio Braido
Department of Internal Medicine,
Genoa University, Genoa, Italy
fulvio.braido@unige.it

Giorgio Walter Canonica
Department of Internal Medicine, Allergy
and Respiratory Diseases Clinic,
University of Genova Maragliano
Pavilion, S Martino Hospital Largo
R. Benzi 10, 16132 Genoa, Italy
canonica@unige.it

Atsushi Fukunaga, MD
Department of Clinical Molecular
Medicine, Division of Dermatology,
Kobe University Graduate School of
Medicine, 7-5-1 Kusunoki-cho,
Chuo-ku, Kobe 650-0017, Japan

Jürgen Grabbe
Department of Deruratology, Kantonsspital
Aarau, 5001 Aarau, Switzerland
juergen.grabbe@ksa.ch

Clive E. H. Grattan, MA, MD, FRCP
Department of Dermatology,
Norfolk and Norwich University Hospital,
Norwich NR4 7UY, UK
clive.grattan@nnuh.nhs.uk

M. Greaves
Cutaneous Allergy Clinic, St. Johns
Institute of Dermatology, St. Thomas
Hospital, London SE1 7EH, UK
malcolmgreaves@clinidermsolutions.co.uk

Tatsuya Horikawa, MD
Division of Dermatology,
Department of Clinical Molecular
Medicine, Kobe University Graduate
School of Medicine, 7-5-1 Kusunoki-cho,
Chuo-un, Kobe 650-0017, Japan
thorikaw@med.kobe-u.ac.jp

Frances Lawlor
Dermatology Department, 2nd Floor,
Outpatients Building,
Royal London Hospital, Whitechapel,
E1 1BD London, UK
Urticaria Clinic
St John's Institute of Dermatology
Block 7 South Wing, St Thomas' Hospital,
SE1 7EH London, UK
frances.lawlor@gstt.nhs.uk
frances.lawlor@bartsandthelondon.nhs.uk

Kieron S. Leslie, MBBS, MRCP, DTM&H
Departments of Dermatology,
University of California, 1701 Divisadero
Street, San Francisco, CA 94115, USA
lesliek@derm.ucsf.edu

M. Magerl
Depatment of Dermatology and Allergy,
Allergy-Centre-Charité Charité –
Universitätsmedizin BerlinCharitéplatz
1D, 10117 Berlin, Germany
markus.magerl@charite.de

Marcus Maurer, MD
Department of Dermatology and Allergy,
Allergie-Centrum-Charité/ECARF,
Charité - Universitätsmedizin Berlin,
Charitéplatz 1, 10117 Berlin, Germany
marcus.maurer@charite.de

M. Metz
Department of Dermatology and Allergy,
Allergy-Centre-Charité, Charité-
Universitätsmedizin Berlin, Charitéplatz 1,
10117 Berlin
martin.metz@charite.de

Chikako Nishigori, MD
Department of Clinical Molecular
Medicine, Division of Dermatology,
Kobe University Graduate School of
Medicine, 7-5-1 Kusunoki-cho,
Chuo-ku, Kobe 650-0017, Japan

Lluís Puig
Department of Dermatology, Hospital
Santa Creu i Sant Pau., Universitat
Autònoma de Barcelona, Sant Antoni
Maria Claret 167, 08025 Barcelona, Spain
lpuig@santpau.cat

Ruth A. Sabroe, FRCP, MD
Barnsley Hospital NHS Foundation
Trust, Gawber Road, Barnsley S75 2EP,
UK
rsabroe@doctors.org.uk

Kanade Shinkai, MD, PhD
Departments of Dermatology and
Dermapathology,
University of California, San Francisco,
1701 Divisadero Street, San Francisco,
CA 94115, USA
shinkaik@derm.ucsf.edu

Bettina Wedi, MD, PhD, Prof.
Department of Dermatology and
Allergology, Hannover Medical
University, Ricklinger Strasse 5,
30449 Hannover, Germany
wedi.bettina@mh-hannover.de

Torsten Zuberbier
Department of Dermatology
and Allergy, Allergy Centre Charité,
Charité – Universitätsmedizin Berlin,
Charitéplatz 1, 10117 Berlin,
Germany
torsten.zuberbier@charite.de

History of Urticaria

1

M Greaves

Core Messages

- The beginning of the twentieth century ushered in the era of molecular medicine, eventually leading to unravelling of the molecular and immunological basis of urticaria.
- The mast cell and its histamine content remain central to the pathophysiology of the pruritic wheal in most forms of urticaria, and the synthesis, storage, regulation of release of histamine as well as molecular characterisation of its receptors are becoming well understood.
- The challenge of the past 50 years has been to understand the causation of the promiscuous activation of dermal and mucosal mast cells in idiopathic chronic urticaria and angioedema.
- The discovery in the 1980s of autoreactivity in the serum of some patients with chronic urticaria (the autologous serum skin test) was a major step forward and prompted attempts to identify and characterise this activity.
- The subsequent finding in chronic urticaria of specific complement-dependent autoantibodies, which release histamine and other mediators from mast cells and basophils via dimerisation of their high affinity IgE receptors, has stimulated intense interest in the multifactorial modes of activation of mast cells and basophils in this disorder.
- Antihistamines, discovered in the 1940s, remain the cornerstone of treatment of most types of urticaria. Although recent derivative ("second-generation") compounds manifest greatly refined properties, they are often only moderately effective.
- New therapeutic approaches "round the corner" include bradykinin B2 antagonists (for angioedema) and the anti-IgE immunobiologic omalizumab.

M. Greaves
Cutaneous Allergy Clinic, St. Johns Institute of Dermatology, St. Thomas Hospital, London SE1 7EH, UK
e-mail: malcolmgreaves@clinidermsolutions.co.uk

T. Zuberbier et al. (eds.), *Urticaria and Angioedema*,
DOI: 10.1007/978-3-540-79048-8_1, © Springer Verlag Berlin Heidelberg 2010

1.1 Introduction

The history of urticaria divides itself conveniently into the early, clinically descriptive, and later pathophysiological eras. Much has been written on the early history of urticaria as a clinical entity, from Hippocrates in the fourth century BC to Heberden and Willan at the end of the eighteenth century AD. For useful accounts of urticaria in early Western writings, the reader is referred to publications by Czarnetzki [1] and Humphreys [2] and the ESHDV Special Annual Lecture entitled "The History of Urticaria and Angioedema" delivered by the late Lennart Juhlin in 2000, a transcript of which is available online. However, in the last hundred years, a dramatic increase in the understanding of the cellular and molecular basis of some common forms of urticaria took place, the foundations for which were laid down by pioneers in the latter years of the nineteenth century and in the early and later twentieth century. This period is the focus of the present account, which attempts to reveal to the reader a historical perspective on "how we got to where we are" today in urticaria.

1.2 The Cellular and Molecular Basis of Urticaria: First Steps

Although the mast cell ("mastzellen") was discovered by Paul Ehrlich in 1877 [3], that it is the principal source and repository of tissue histamine (including the skin) was not appreciated until the seminal work of Riley and West was published in a series of papers in the 1950s. The correlation between histamine levels and mast cell content of skin of several species is well described in several publications summarised by Riley [4]. Histamine was discovered in 1906 by Dale in extracts of ergot [5] and he described all the important actions of histamine except for stimulation of gastric acid secretion. Dale also established the famous "Dale criteria," which should be fulfilled by a mediator deemed to be responsible for a given inflammatory response. Indeed, these criteria are only completely satisfied by histamine in the pruritic wheals of urticaria – hence we have previously designated histamine as the "quintessential mediator" [6].

It was Lewis who first delineated the potency of histamine as a mediator of whealing in human skin [7]. Lewis showed that, in low dosage, histamine could produce central whealing (vasopermeability) redness (vasodilation) and a surrounding bright red axon reflex flare (Lewis's triple response) characteristic of the urticarial wheal. Curiously, in all his intensive studies of actions of histamine in skin, he never once mentions itching! We now know that, in addition to itching (and pain), intracutaneous injection of histamine can also cause alloknesis (perception of itching in response to local nonpruritic stimuli such as fine touch or even temperature change) [8]. These vascular effects are receptor-mediated and involve two subclasses of histamine receptors, H1 and H2, both of which were cloned and sequenced in the early 1990s [9, 10]. Histamine-induced itching is served by H1 receptors. First evidence of the effectiveness of H1 antagonists in the treatment of urticaria emerged in the late 1940s [11, 12]. Recently described and characterised H4 receptors and their antagonists [13] are currently under scrutiny regarding possible relevance to urticaria and its management. That histamine is released in lesional skin of chronic urticaria has been demonstrated repeatedly in skin tissue fluid, and more recently by skin microdialysis technology [14, 15]. However, histamine, although playing a significant role, is clearly not the only mediator, especially in chronic urticaria and this supposition is supported by kinetic studies [16].

1.3 The Enigma of Chronic "Idiopathic" Urticaria

The problem of how, in urticaria, the dermal mast cell is prompted to relieve itself of its burden of histamine and other mediators has puzzled investigators in the post Second World War era. The discovery and characterisation of the "reaginic" IgE immunoglobulin by Ishizaka [17] enabled elucidation of the relatively uncomplicated acute allergic urticaria, which could be explained by a straightforward immediate (Gell and Coombs type I reaction) [18] between dermal mast cell-bound IgE and specific allergen leading to release of histamine and other mast cell-derived mediators. However, the aetiology and pathogenesis of chronic "idiopathic" urticaria (CIU) remained obscure and even in the twenty-first century there remain numerous unanswered questions. Why do the dermal mast cells degranulate explosively in a seemingly random way with no evident triggering factor?

In the 1960s and 1970s, attempts were made, mainly in Europe, to popularise the role of common food additives, colouring agents and preservatives such as tartrazine, sodium benzoate, and antioxidants as aetiological agents in CIU. Protagonists of this theory included Juhlin, Doeglas and Warner [19–21]. Complex exclusion diets were devised and successes were claimed. Some of these regimes did include challenge tests, but were not adequately controlled and the reproducibility of apparent positive reactions was not investigated. Latterly, this approach has been revived and refined, food additives now being described as "pseudoallergens" [22], further successes being claimed following use of pseudoallergen-free diets in CIU, but this issue, which was reviewed in more detail recently [23], remains controversial.

Foci of infections are always liable to be invoked to explain otherwise inexplicable relapses in any chronic diseases, and chronic urticaria is no exception. The literature contains numerous usually anecdotal accounts of patients with severe chronic and recalcitrant urticaria who made a dramatic recovery following removal of an infected gallbladder/tooth, or treatment of an infected sinus or urinary tract. The 1980s saw the emergence of a new putative microbial culprit – Helicobacter pylori. Because of its ubiquity, especially in European populations, it was frequently found in patients with CIU. When patients with Helicobacter were treated, some got better both from the infection and from the urticaria. Although carefully controlled studies have not substantiated an aetiological relationship between H pylori and urticaria despite its frequency in these patients [24], a more indirect role in the pathogenesis has been proposed [25].

The notion that antibodies may be causative in CIU is an old one. As long ago as 1962, Rorsman, a Swedish dermatologist, reported the striking basopenia in chronic urticaria and remarked on its absence in physical urticarias. He also pointed out that "In cases where the basopenia is marked it appears probable that antigen–antibody reactions ... bring about degranulation of basophil leukocytes" [26]. Over 20 years later [27], we noted the impaired histamine release evoked by anti-IgE in basophils from patients with CIU. In 1988, Gruber et al. found that more than 50% of patients with cold urticaria, CIU and urticarial vasculitis had IgG autoantibodies directed against IgE [28]. There was also indirect evidence arising from the strong association between autoimmune thyroid disease and CIU [29]. The HLA class 11 DRB1*04 alleles were increased in frequency in CIU consistent with a possible role for autoimmunity in CIU [30]. However, at this juncture there was no convincing evidence that any autoantibodies found in CIU were anything more than passive bystanders in the pathogenesis of this disorder.

Against this background, an important observation was made in 1986 by Grattan [31]. He demonstrated that the serum of some but not all patients with CIU would cause whealing when reinjected intracutaneously in an autologous fashion into the same patient's clinically uninvolved skin. This finding greatly encouraged attempts to identify circulating vasoactive factors in the blood of CIU patients [32, 33]. As had previously been suspected by earlier writers [26, 28], the culprit turned out to be a functional, histamine-releasing autoantibody – at least in some patients. Hide et al. in 1993 and subsequently Fiebiger et al. and Tong et al. found that in 30–50% of patients with CIU, a circulating histamine-releasing factor with the characteristics of an IgG anti-FcεR1 autoantibody was demonstrable in serum [34–37]. Indirect evidence as well as successful passive transfer [38] supported the view that these autoantibodies are the cause of the whealing in those patients that have them. Although "autoimmune urticaria" has yet to justify, in a strict sense, its designation as an autoimmune disease (there is no animal model), these advances have for the first time put the investigation and treatment of chronic urticaria on a sound scientific basis. Lack of a convenient specific and sensitive screening test for autoimmune urticaria remains the main drawback to further progress.

1.4 Treatment of Urticaria: Antihistamines

Fortunately, most patients with chronic urticaria, whatever the cause, can be effectively managed by H1 antihistamines. These were first characterised by Bovet and Staub [39], a discovery which was, in part, responsible for conferment of the Nobel Prize on Bovet in 1957. Their use in treatment of chronic urticaria was explored intensively after the end of the First World War [11, 12]. O'Leary and Farber, referring in 1947 to diphenhydramine [11] stated that it is effective in chronic urticaria and also pointed out that it "is not a potent antipruritic drug" – a view that present-day clinicians will echo in respect of its present-day successors. These early "first-generation" antihistamines, though carrying a baggage of annoying rather than serious side effects, are still very much in use today by urticaria sufferers. Although initially believed to be competitive antagonists of histamine at the H1 receptor, all currently available H1 antihistamines are now considered to behave as inverse agonists – that is, they downregulate and stabilise the constitutively activated state of the H1 receptor [40]. H2 histamine receptors are also expressed by human skin blood vessels [41] and the possibility was entertained that combination of H2 receptor antagonists (e.g. cimetidine) with first-generation H1 antihistamines would have a "sparing" effect on the latter, thus mitigating the unwanted effects of H1 antihistamines. Although some benefits were established for use of this combination [42], they were small and in any case their use was largely superseded by the advent of second-generation antihistamines.

Second-generation H1 antihistamines, as defined by Simons [43], are essentially H1 antihistamines with low or non-sedating properties at therapeutic dosages. Many of these are active metabolites or enantiomers of first-generation compounds. Their usage over the past 15 years in chronic urticaria, especially as daytime treatment, has greatly improved the quality of life of otherwise severely handicapped sufferers [44–47]. However, they are less effective in relieving whealing than itching in urticaria and sedative first-generation antihistamines still have a place in the management of nocturnal pruritus in urticaria sufferers. Combination of montelukast, a leucotriene inhibitor, with an H1 antihistamine has been advocated, but results have been variable [48]. The cloning and sequencing of the H1 receptor in 1991 [9, 49] has laid the foundation for emergence of a truly new "third generation" of anthistamines for clinicians and patients alike to look forward to.

Future developments in the diagnosis and management of urticaria have also been greatly encouraged by the recent establishment of European Guidelines for definition, classification, diagnosis and management of urticaria [50, 51]. These should also give much needed help to clinicians faced with investigation and treatment of urticaria.

1.5 Take Home Pearls

- The autologous serum skin test established that in patients with chronic "idiopathic" urticaria, the causation was endogenous rather than due to external factors such as food allergy or pseudoallergy, and "focal infection."
- In some patients, this endogenous activity turned out to be attributable to specific autoantibodies (autoimmune urticaria), which promiscuously activate dermal mast cells and basophils and this has led to advent of immunotherapy (e.g. cyclosporine) in selected patients.
- The "cause" of chronic urticaria is, however, multifactorial and other factors such as dysregulation of intracellular signal transduction in dermal mast cells and basophils are likely to be important in other patients.
- However, H1 antihistamines remain the mainstay of treatment and recent refinements have greatly improved the effectiveness and tolerability of these compounds.
- As knowledge of the pathomechanisms of urticaria advances, novel treatments are appearing, including the anti-IgE monoclonal omalizumab and anti-cytokines such as anti-TNF-α.

References

1. Czarnetzki BM. History of urticaria. Int J Dermatol. 1989;28:52–7
2. Humphreys F. Major landmarks in the history of urticarial disorders. Int J Dermatol. 1997;36:793–96
3. Ehrlich P. Beitrage zur Kenntnis der Anilinfarbungen und ihrer in der Verwendung mikroskopischen Technik. Arch Mikr-Anat. 1877;13:263–77
4. Riley JF. The mast cells. Chapter 16: Mast cells and histamine in the skin. Edinburgh: E&S Livingstone, 1959. p. 144–59
5. Dale HH. On some physiological actions of ergot. J Physiol. 1906;34:163–206
6. Greaves MW, Sabroe RA. Histamine: the quintessential mediator. J Dermatol. 1996;23:735–40
7. Lewis T. The blood vessels of the human skin and their responses. London: Shaw; 1927
8. Simone DA, Alreja M, La Motte RH. Psychophysical studies of the itch sensation and itchy skin (alloknesis) produced by intacutaneous injection of histamine. Somatosens Mot Res. 1991;8:271–79
9. Le Coniat M, Traiffort E, Ruat M, Arrang J-M, Berger R. Chromosomal localisation of the human histamine H1 receptor gene. Hum Genet. 1994;94:186–8
10. Gantz I, Schaffer M, DelValle J, et al Molecular cloning of the gene encoding the histamine H2 receptor. Proc Nat Acad Sci USA. 1991;88:429–33
11. O'Leary PA, Farber EM. Benadryl in the treatment of certain diseases of the skin. J Am Med Assoc 1947;134:1010–13
12. Bain WA, Hellier FF, Warin RP. Some aspects of the action of histamine antagonists. Lancet 1948;2:964–69
13. Fung-Leung W-P, Thurmond RL, Ling P, Karlsson L. Histamie H4 antagonists: the new antihistamines ? Curr Opin Invest New Drugs. 2004;5:1174–80
14. Kaplan AP, Horakova, Z, Katz SI. Assessment of tissue fluid histamine levels in patients with urticaria. J Allergy Clin Immunol. 1978;61:350–54
15. Okahara K, Murakami T, Yamamoto S, Yata N. Skin microdialysis. Detection of in vivo histamine release in cutaneous allergic reactions. Skin Pharmacol. 1995;8:113–18
16. Cook J, Shuster S. Histamine wheal formation and absorption in Man. Br J Pharmacol. 1980; 69:579–85
17. Ishizaka, K, Ishizaka T, Hornbrook MM. Physicochemical properties of reaginic antibody: correlation of reaginic antibody with γE antibody. J Immunol. 1966;97:840–53
18. Gell PGH, Coombs RR. Clinical aspects of immunology. Oxford: Blackwell; 1963. p. 317–20
19. Michaelsson G, Juhlin L. Urticaria inuced by preservatives and dye additives in food and drugs. Br J Dermatol. 1973;88:525–32
20. Doeglas HMG. Reactions t aspirin and food additives in patients with chronic urticaria including the physical urticarias. Br J Dermatol. 1975;93:135–44
21. Supramanian G, Warner JO. Artificial food additive intolerance in patients with angioedema and urticaria. Lancet 1986;2:907–10
22. Zuberbier T, Chantraine-Hess S, Hartman K, Czarnetzki BM. Pseudoallergen free diet in the treatment of chronic urticaria – a prospective study. Acta Dermato-vener (Stockh). 1995;75:484–87
23. Greaves M. Food Intolerance in urticaria and angioedema and urticarial vasculitis. *In* Food Allergy and Intolerance 2nd Ed. 2002; Brostoff J, Challacombe S, Eds, Philadelphia: WB Saunders. P623–69
24. Burova GP, Mallet AI, Greaves MW. Is *Helicobacter pylori* a cause of chronic urticaria. Br J Dermatol. 1998;139 Suppl 51:42
25. Greaves MW. Chronic idiopathic urticaria and *Helicobacter pylori*: not directly related – but could there be a link? ACI Int 2001;13:23–6
26. Rorsman H. Basophilic leucopenia in different forms of urticaria. Acta Allergologica. 1962;17: 168–84
27. Greaves MW, Plummer VM, Mc Laughlan P, Stanworth DR. Serum and cell bound IgE in chronic urticaria. Clin Allergy. 1974;4:265–71

28. Gruber BL, Baeza ML, Marchese MJ, et al Prevalence and functional role of anti-IgE autoantibodies in urticarial syndromes. J Invest Dermatol. 1988;90:213–17
29. Leznoff A, Sussman GL. Syndrome of idiopathic urticaria and angioedema with thyroid autoimmunity: a study of 90 patients. J Allergy Clin Immunol. 1989;84:66–71
30. O'Donnell BF, O'Neill CM, Francis DM, et al Human leucocyte class 11 associations in chronic idiopathic urticaria. Br J Dermatol. 1999;140:853–88
31. Grattan CEH, Wallington TB, Warin RP, et al A serological mediator in chronic idiopathic urticaria – a clinical immunological and histological evaluation. Br J Dermatol. 1986;114: 583–90
32. Claveau J, Lavoie A, Brunet C, et al Chronic idiopathic urticaria: possible contribution of histamine –releasing factor to pathogenesis. J Allergy Clin Immunol. 1993;92:132–37
33. MacDonald SM, Rafnar T, Langdon J, Lichtenstein SM. Molecular identification of an IgE-dependent histamine releasing factor. Science 1995;269:688–70
34. Hide M, Francis DM, Grattan CEH, et al Autoantibodies against the high affinity IgE receptor as a cause for histamine release in chronic urticaria. N Eng J Med. 1993;328:1599–604
35. Nimii N, Francis DM, Kermani F, et al Dermal mast cell activation by autoantibodies against the high affinity IgE receptor in chronic urticaria. J Invest Dermatol. 1996;106:1001–10
36. Fiebiger E, Maurer D, Holub H, et al Serum IgG autoantibodies directed against the alpha – chain of FcεR1; a selective marker and pathogenetic factor for a distinct subset of chronic urticaria patients. J Clin Invest. 1995;96:2606–12
37. Tong LJ, Balakrishnan G, Kochan JP, et al Assessment of autoimmunity in patients with chronic urticaria. J Allergy Clin Immunol. 1997;99:461–65
38. Grattan CEH, Francis DM. Autoimmune urticaria. Adv Dermatol. 1999;15:311–40
39. Staub A, Bovet D. Actions de la thymoethyl-diethylamine (929F) et des ethersphenoliques sur le choc anaphylactique du cobaye. CR Soc Biol. 1937;128:818–25
40. Leurs R, Church MK, Taglialatela M. H1 antihistamines: inverse agonism. Anti – inflammatory effects and cardiac effects. Clin Exp Allergy. 2002;32:489–98
41. Marks R, Greaves MW. Vascular reactions to histamine and compound 48/80 in human skin: suppression by an H2 receptor blocking agent. Br J Clin Pharmacol. 1977;4:367–69
42. Bleehen SS, Thomas SE, Greaves MW, et al Cimetidine and chlorpheniramine in the treatment of chronic idiopathic urticaria. Br J Dermatol. 1987;117:81–8
43. Simons FER, Simons KJ. The pharmacology and use of H1 receptor antagonist drugs. N Eng J Med. 1994;330:1663–70
44. Breneman DL. Cetirizine versus hydroxyzine and placebo in chronic idiopathic urticaria. Ann Pharmacother. 1996;30:1075–79
45. Finn AF, Kaplan AP, Fretwell R, et al A double-blind placebo-controlled trial of fexofenadine hydrochloride in the treatment of chronic idiopathic urticaria. J Allergy Clin Immunol. 1999; 104:1071–78
46. Paul E, Berth-Jones J, Ortonne J-P, Stern M. Fexofenadine hydrochloride in the treatment of chronic idiopathic urticaria: a placebo – controlled parallel group, dose ranging study. J Dermatol Treat. 1998;9:143–49
47. Zuberbier T, Munzberger C, Haustein U, et al Double – blind crossover study of high dose cetirizine in cholinergic urticaria. Dermatology 1996;193:324–37
48. Di Lorenzo G, Pacor ML, Mansueto P, et al Randomised placebo-controlled trial comparing deslratidine and montelukast in monotherapy and desloratidine plus montelukast in combined therapy for chronic idiopathic urticaria. J Allergy Clin Immunol. 2004;114:619–25
49. Yamashita M, Fukui H, Sugama K, et al Expression cloning of a cDNA encoding the bovine histamine H1 receptor. Proc Natl Acad Sci USA. 1991;88:115–19
50. Zuberbier T, Bindslev-Jensen C, Canonica W, et al EAACI/GA²LEN/EDF guideline: definition, classification and diagnosis of urticaria. Allergy 2006;61:321–31
51. Zuberbier T, Bindslev-Jensen C, Canonica W, et al EAACI/GA²LEN guideline: management of urticaria. Allergy 2006;61:316–20

Aetiopathogenesis of Urticaria

2

Clive E. H. Grattan

Core Messages

- Urticaria is a disease with diverse clinical presentations and aetiologies
- The cutaneous mast cell is the primary effector cell in most patterns of urticaria
- Histamine is the most important preformed mediator in mast cells. It mediates itch, weal and flare
- Leukotrienes may also be important in pseudoallergic reactions
- Bradykinin is responsible for angio-oedema in patients with C1 esterase inhibitor deficiency and in patients on angiotensin converting enzyme inhibitors
- Mast cell degranulation may be due to immunological stimuli activating the high affinity IgE receptor (FcεRI) or non-immunological stimuli, such as opiates
- Activation of FcεRI may be through allergen cross-linking of specific IgE bound to the receptor (Type I hypersensitivity) or IgE autoantibodies binding the receptor directly or IgE itself
- Type I reactions may be the cause of acute urticaria but not chronic disease. Functional autoantibodies can be demonstrated in about 50% of patients with ordinary spontaneous chronic urticaria
- The role for inflammatory cells in urticarial lesions needs further investigation

Urticaria is defined clinically by swellings of the integument that resolve completely within hours or days. Superficial skin swellings, known as weals, usually begin as sharply defined pale plaques of variable size with a surrounding red flare. They nearly always itch intensely before changing from pale to pink, spreading outwards and becoming more diffuse before fading. The deeper swellings of angio-oedema are predominantly located in the loose connective tissue below the skin and the mucosa. They tend to be pale and painful and last longer than weals. Within this basic clinical definition of urticaria exists a wide spectrum of presentations that can usually be grouped into patterns on the strength of

C. E. H. Grattan
Department of Dermatology, Norfolk and Norwich University Hospital, Norwich NR4 7UY, UK
e-mail: clive.grattan@nnuh.nhs.uk

T. Zuberbier et al. (eds.), *Urticaria and Angioedema*,
DOI: 10.1007/978-3-540-79048-8_2, © Springer Verlag Berlin Heidelberg 2010

clinical features. These patterns may help clinicians to investigate and manage individual patients appropriately, but in themselves, do not define aetiology or pathogenesis, which often remain poorly understood and difficult to demonstrate. The aim of this chapter is to walk backwards from the patient to the pathways that mediate the events of urticaria, illustrating the diversity and overlap that may occur and to speculate a little on some potential explanations for the "idiopathic" aspects of this complex disease.

It is now increasingly accepted that many, if not most, patients with chronic continuous urticaria have an endogenous rather than an exogenous cause of their illness. In addition to somehow acquiring this primary endogenous tendency to develop spontaneous urticaria, clinical experience indicates that there is a wide range of secondary external aggravating factors that can bring out weals and angio-oedema, which influence the day-to-day variability of the illness. These include localised heat, pressure, friction, some medicines (especially non-steroidal anti-inflammatory drugs, NSAIDs), dietary pseudoallergens, alcohol, stress and mild infections. In acute urticaria, an identifiable exogenous cause (infectious, allergic or pseudoallergic) may be found [1] but many cases remain unexplained despite evaluation and some of these will evolve into chronic disease. Since the cutaneous mast cell is the key effector cell of acute and chronic urticaria, it is very likely that the mediator pathways are similar even though the initiating cause may be different. In acute and chronic urticaria the eruption of weals and angio-oedema is mainly spontaneous, unlike the physical urticarias, in which lesions are induced by a unique physical trigger or triggers. The main role of the clinician is to identify this trigger since the activity of the urticaria can, in theory, be reduced by avoiding the stimulus. This does not address what has caused urticaria in the first place, which essentially remains unknown, although information from passive transfer studies implicating immunoglobulin E in cold, cholinergic, solar and dermographism over 3 decades ago has not been explored further. It is likely that differences will emerge between the mediators of induced and spontaneous urticaria as more becomes known about the local mediator and cytokine profiles in lesional and non-lesional skin. This is especially true of urticarial vasculitis, which should be considered as a pattern of small vessel vasculitis even though it is often included in classifications of urticaria because of the similarity in the appearance of the skin lesions with spontaneous weals. Hereditary angio-oedema, due to mutations in the gene for C1 esterase inhibitor on chromosome 11q11 resulting in complement consumption and kinin formation, and the urticarial autoinflammatory syndromes, defined by mutations of *CIAS*1 on chromosome 1q44 resulting in activation of the NALP3 inflammasome complex [2] with the generation of interleukin-1β and -18, illustrate the fundamental differences in aetiopathogenesis that exist between different clinical patterns of urticaria, and the implications for investigation and management that flow from this.

2.1 Lessons from Histopathology

The histology of urticaria may seem bland and non-specific but the pathological features complement and extend what can be deduced from the clinical features. The intensity and depth of dermal oedema depends on the timing and depth of the swelling, favouring the papillary dermis in weals and the deep dermis and subcutis in angio-oedema. The oedema fluid originates from postcapillary venules rather than arterioles. Lumina of individual vessels may be dilated and the integrity of their linings compromised due to transient contraction and separation of endothelial cells. High molecular weight proteins, including immunoglobulins, are then able to pass temporarily from the lumina to the interstitium until the leak repairs. Fluid is removed via lymphatic vessels that become dilated early during weal formation. Although small blood vessels are functionally impaired by these events, they are not permanently damaged, unlike the changes that are seen in small vessel vasculitis where the postcapillary venules are disrupted to the point of necrosis, leading to passive extravasation of red cells in addition to plasma proteins and recruitment of inflammatory cells. Morphology of the endothelial changes can be best appreciated on semi-thin sections or ultrastructural examination. Inflammatory infiltrates are initially perivascular as leucocytes are recruited actively from the circulation by upregulation of adhesion molecules under the influence of chemokines and then become more diffusely distributed. The qualitative nature and quantitative intensity of the infiltrates has not been studied closely in relation to clinically defined patterns of urticaria but biopsies taken from patients with a diagnostic label of chronic urticaria have shown a spectrum of changes ranging from mild mononuclear perivascular infiltrates to full-blown changes of small vessel vasculitis with numerous neutrophils and eosinophils in a minority [3]. This diversity probably reflects a lack of definition of clinical patterns and the severity of urticaria at the time of biopsy but may also depend on the timing of biopsy in relation to the onset of the lesion. Accurate timing of spontaneous weals is always problematic but it does appear that acute inflammatory cells predominate in the early stages of wheal formation and that mononuclear cells follow later. More neutrophils and eosinophils were present in lesions over 12 h than below 4 h in biopsies of spontaneous weals of chronic urticaria patients [4, 5]. This may explain why the "neutrophilic" pattern of urticaria may be seen in patients with wide-ranging clinical patterns from cold urticaria to acute spontaneous urticaria [6]. Lesional biopsies of patients with chronic "idiopathic" urticaria showed a Th0 cytokine profile [7]. There were no significant differences in the number of inflammatory cells or the cytokine pattern between patients with and without histamine-releasing autoantibodies. With the exception of an increased number of activated eosinophils in 12 h + biopsies of urticaria with functional autoantibodies compared with urticaria without [4, 5], the deep mixed infiltrates or delayed pressure urticaria and the leucocytoclasia with red cell extravasation that define urticarial vasculitis, it is generally true that the qualitative and quantitative features of inflammatory infiltrates do not help define a specific pathogenesis or aetiology for an individual patient.

2.2
A Central Role for the Mast Cell

Central to all these observations is the mast cell. Spontaneous and induced physical urticarias would not happen without them. Early studies using conventional histochemical granule stains appeared to show that they were increased in urticaria lesions [8] when compared with healthy control skin but a later study using tryptase and chymase as a marker showed no difference [9]. This discrepancy might be the result of peripheral blood basophil migration into lesions [10] since basophil granules stain similarly to mast cells but contain little or no tryptase. What is established from functional studies using the mast cell liberators codeine [11] and the experimental degranulation agent, Compound 48/80, is that mast cells of urticaria patients release their contents more readily than mast cells of healthy controls and this is borne out by the rapid wealing response of the physical urticarias when challenged by the appropriate stimulus. Of the pre-formed and newly synthesised mediators released at the time of mast cell degranulation, histamine and the cysteinyl-leukotrienes LTC_4,D_4,E_4 appear to be most relevant to urticaria pathogenesis. Specific roles for heparin, tryptase and chymase remain unclear but a mast cell stabilising effect for heparin (in addition to its known anticoagulant properties) is suggested by the observation that addition of heparin to whole blood can prevent in vitro release of histamine from basophils and abrogate the weal response seen on re-injection of sera from patients with autoimmune urticaria [12].

2.2.1 Mast Cell Mediators of Urticaria

2.2.1.1 Histamine

Binding of histamine H_1 receptors on small cutaneous blood vessels mediates vasopermeability and vasodilatation. It also mediates itch through stimulation of cutaneous nociceptors and the surrounding flare by antidromic stimulation of local C-fibre networks. The flare response is mediated by substance P release from cutaneous nerve endings rather than histamine [13]. Stimulation of H_2 receptors on cutaneous blood vessels is also responsible for vasodilatation and vasopermeability within the weal but not itch or flare. Effects of histamine on the cellular immune system have been demonstrated [14], but their relevance to urticaria is uncertain.

2.2.1.2 Cysteinyl Leukotrienes

The cysteinyl leukotrienes may contribute to vasopermeability and vasodilatation in urticaria but are secondary in importance to histamine. Synthesis of LTC_4,D_4,E_4 by mast cells at the time of degranulation and subsequently by infiltrating basophils and eosinophils may be a factor in the prolongation of urticaria weals in some types of urticaria, particularly aspirin-sensitive urticaria, autoimmune urticaria and delayed pressure urticaria. It is thought that aspirin and other non-selective NSAIDs may activate mast cells indirectly by inhibiting formation of prostaglandin E_2 (PGE_2) via cyclo-oxygenase (COX) for which there is some evidence of an inhibitory effect on immunological mast cell activation [15] (Fig. 2.1). Selective inhibitors of inducible COX-2 are less likely to exacerbate aspirin-sensitive

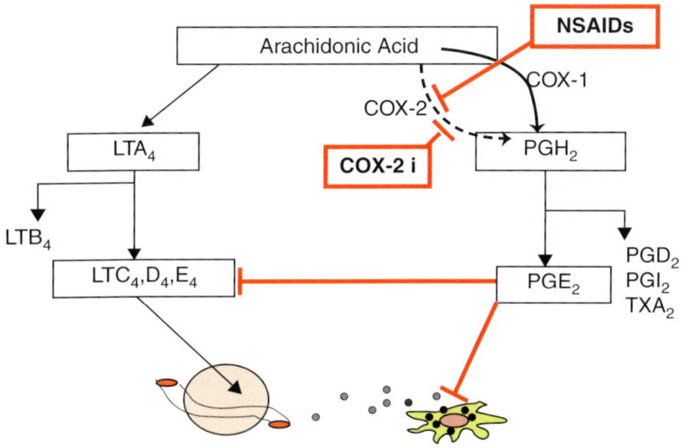

Fig. 2.1 Inhibition of the cyclo-oxygenase (COX) pathway by non-selective NSAIDS results in diversion of arachidonic acid metabolism from prostaglandins to leukotrienes. PGE_2 normally has an inhibitory action on immunological mast cell degranulation and cysteinyl leukotriene production. Reduced PGE_2 formation has a permissive effect on immunological mast cell degranulation that is not seen with selective COX-2 inhibitors

urticaria than non-selective COX-1 and -2 inhibitors since PGE_2 production by the constitutively expressed COX-1 isoform is not affected. Evidence of thrombin generation in citrated plasma of chronic urticaria patients was related to chronic urticaria severity and injection of autologous citrated plasma yielded a higher proportion of positive skin tests than autologous serum [16] suggesting that coagulation factors may enhance vascular permeability or induce mast cell degranulation.

2.3 Involvement of Other Inflammatory Cells in Urticaria

Although the cutaneous mast cell is the primary effector cell of the early phase of urticaria, eosinophils, basophils and lymphocytes almost certainly play a significant role afterwards in the evolution of weals and angio-oedema. Eosinophils contain toxic granules including major basic protein (MBP) and eosinophil cationic protein (ECP) that are released on activation. MPB can degranulate mast cells non-immunologically. Basophils are thought to migrate into weals of chronic urticaria [17] and probably perpetuate the inflammatory oedema by releasing histamine and leukotrienes. No specific role for polymorphonuclear neutrophils has been identified but it is possible that they are involved with oxygen-free radical formation. There is some evidence for oxidative stress being important in the lesional skin of patients with chronic “idiopathic” urticaria [55] but the antioxidant activity in plasma and erythrocytes was similar to that of healthy controls [18]. Studies of skin lymphocyte populations have shown a Th0 phenotype [7]. The contribution of lesional skin lymphocytes to urticaria pathogenesis is uncertain but upregulation of immunoreactivity for interleukin-3 (IL-3) and tumour necrosis factor alpha (TNF-α) was seen in perivascular cells in the upper dermis of patients with acute urticaria and delayed pressure urticaria, but not chronic urticaria [19]. CD40L expression was higher on activated circulating T-cells in chronic urticaria than healthy controls implying that co-stimulatory signals for B-cell activation are upregulated [20]. Bcl-2 protein expression on blood B and T cells was enhanced in severe chronic urticaria, consistent with their prolonged survival and proliferation [21], although peripheral blood lymphocyte numbers were consistently lower in untreated active chronic urticaria patients than controls on automated differential counts [17].

2.4 Urticaria Not Implicating the Mast Cell (Non-histaminergic)

Bradykinin generated by the action of kallikrein on kininogen appears to be the primary mediator of hereditary angio-oedema (Fig. 2.2). Evidence for generation of C2 kinin by the action of plasmin on C2b in humans is poor. C1 esterase inhibitor prevents initiation of the intrinsic coagulation pathway by activated Hageman factor (XIIa), plasmin formation, the classical pathway of complement activation and the kallikrein–kininogen–kinin system. Kininase II (also known as angiotensin converting enzyme) inhibition by angio-

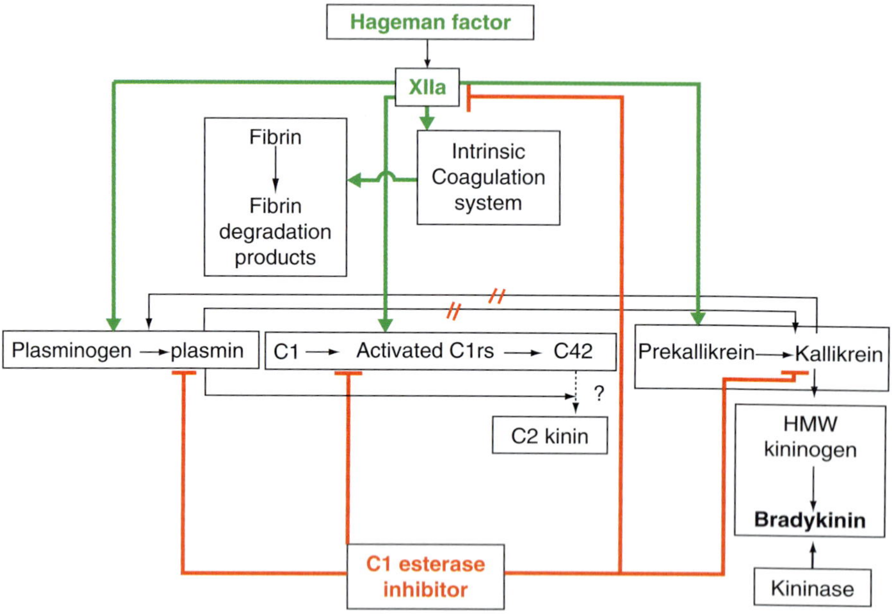

Fig. 2.2 Stimulation of Hageman factor XII activates the intrinsic coagulation system, generation of plasmin and production of bradykinin by the action of kallikrein on high molecular weight kininogen. There is a complex interconnecting system of feedback loops involving C1 esterase inhibitor, which has a controlling inhibitory influence on the complement, kallikrein, coagulation and fibrinolytic systems

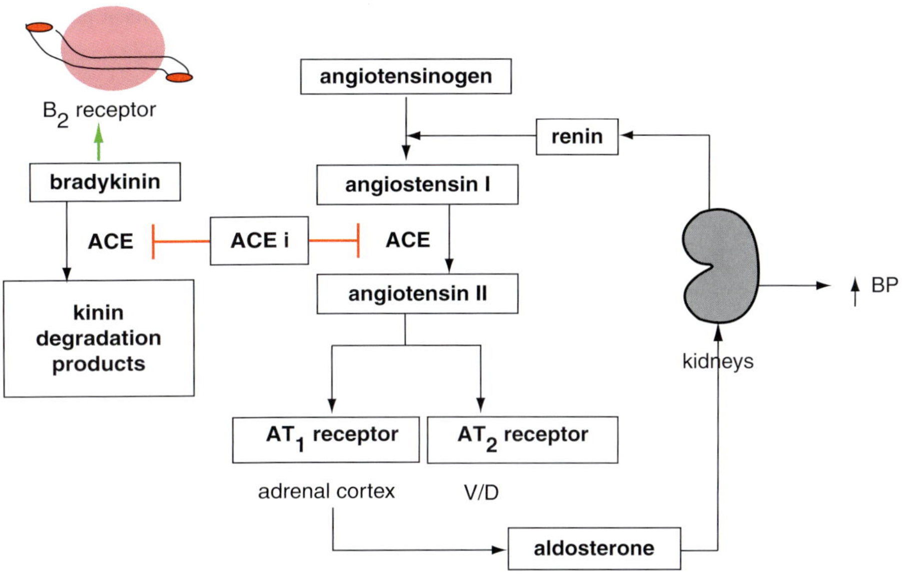

Fig. 2.3 Inhibitors of angiotensin converting enzyme (ACE) block the angiotensin–renin system that controls blood pressure and the breakdown of bradykinin, which may lead to angio-oedema through stimulation of B_2 receptors on blood vessels

tensin converting enzyme inhibitors (ACEI) may result in accumulation of kinins leading to angio-oedema *without* weals but is not a cause of angio-oedema *with* weals (Fig. 2.3). Although, in theory, NSAIDs could result in urticaria due to overproduction of leukotrienes alone, it seems likely that histamine is also involved in NSAID-induced urticaria in view of the beneficial response to antihistamines seen in clinical practice in this group of patients.

2.5 What Causes Mast Cell Mediator Release in the First Place?

Understanding the stimulus for mast cell mediator secretion is the key to diagnosis and appropriately directed management in clinical practice. The stimulus may be immunological, non-immunological or, perhaps, a combination of both in some situations. In reality, it is often not possible to be certain and it is these cases that should be labelled idiopathic. A "guestimate" of the frequency of the aetiologies of urticaria is shown in Table 2.1, but it must be recognised that there may be considerable variation with age, geographical areas and the populations seen by different medical specialties. The commonest cause of anaphylaxis and contact urticaria is allergy, mediated by cross-linking specific IgE on mast cells by an allergen. In contrast, allergy is probably never the cause of chronic continuous

Table 2.1 Estimated order of frequency of different aetiologies of urticaria by clinical pattern in Western Europe

Ordinary (spontaneous) urticaria
Acute: idiopathic > upper respiratory tract infection > allergy > pseudoallergic
Episodic: idiopathic > pseudoallergic > allergy > autoimmune
Chronic: autoimmune > idiopathic > pseudoallergic > chronic infection
Physical urticarias
Triggers are defined by challenge testing but the aetiology is unknown
Angio-oedema without weals
Idiopathic > drug-induced > C1 esterase inhibitor deficiency
Urticarial vasculitis
Idiopathic > immunological > drugs > chronic viral infection
Contact urticaria
Allergic > non-allergic
Autoinflammatory syndromes
Hereditary (cryopyrin associated periodic syndrome) > acquired

urticaria. Here, the stimulus for mast cell degranulation appears to be binding of autoantibodies to the alpha subunit of the high affinity IgE receptor (FcεRIα) or to IgE on cutaneous mast cells and basophils (Fig. 2.4). These functional autoantibodies have been demonstrated in around 50% of patients with the ordinary presentation of chronic urticaria. The incidence of urticaria from exposure to agents that cause mast cell degranulation non-immunologically (known as mast cell liberators) and pseudoallergens without an additional aetiological factor is probably quite low.

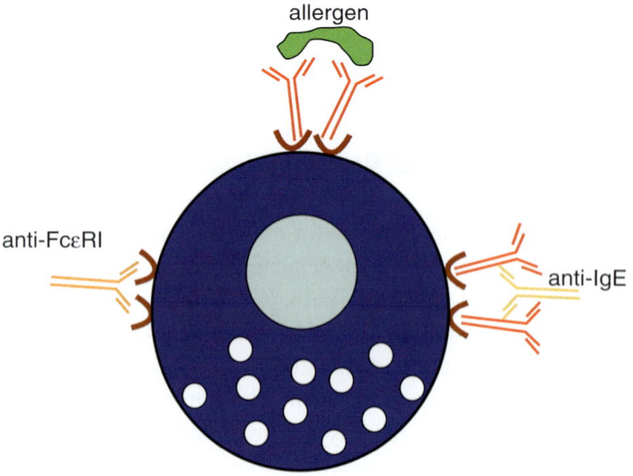

Fig. 2.4 Cross-linking of high affinity IgE receptors (FcεRI) by allergen binding to specific cytophilic IgE, IgE itself or its receptor by functional autoantibodies results in mast cell and basophil degranulation

2.5.1 Immunological Stimuli of Mast Cell Secretion

2.5.1.1 Allergens

Although contact urticaria and anaphylaxis are often due to immediate hypersensitivity reactions, allergy was an uncommon cause of acute urticaria in the setting of a specialist walk-in clinic [1]. Allergic reactions to foods, drugs and blood products usually last for hours or days only, provided the cause is suspected and avoided, whereas acute urticaria initiated by upper respiratory tract viral infections may be continuous for a week or more. Patients presenting with the oral allergy syndrome due to cross-reactivity between foods with homologous proteins in pollens have a form of contact urticaria due to mast cell degranulation from interaction of the relevant food allergen with specific IgE to pollen. The term Food Contact Hypersensitivity Syndrome has recently been proposed to embrace all mucosal food contact urticarial reactions, whether due to cross-reactivity with homologous proteins or not [22].

2.5.1.2 Autoantibodies

There is a considerable body of evidence from different centres on both sides of the Atlantic confirming the presence of functional IgG autoantibodies in adults [23–28] and children with chronic urticaria [29]. In addition to anti-FcεRIα and anti-IgE, autoantibodies have been described against the low affinity IgE receptor (FcεRII) on eosinophils that cause release of MPB which, in turn, may lead to non-immunological degranulation of mast cells [30]. Functional autoantibodies have not been found in patients with cholinergic urticarias, symptomatic dermographism or in healthy controls [31]. Histamine-releasing autoantibodies [54] and chronic urticaria serum-induced upregulation of healthy donor basophil CD63 [32] are reduced by treatment with cyclosporin, but may occasionally be detected in patients who appear to be in clinical remission (probably because they remain at risk of relapse). However, long-term studies looking at the levels of autoantibodies and disease severity have not been undertaken. Debate continues about the importance of functional autoantibodies, which are considered by some to be a secondary event in urticaria pathogenesis rather than a defining feature of autoimmune urticaria. The main reasons for this are threefold: first that non-functional autoantibodies against the FcεRIα and IgE have been found in patients with other autoimmune dermatological diseases [33] and healthy controls [34] by immunoassays (Western blot and ELISA) as well as chronic urticaria; second, that there is still no widely available assay for their detection in clinical practice and third that autoantibody-negative chronic urticaria patients behave similarly in their clinical presentation and response to treatment but tend to be less severe and may respond less well to immunomodulatory therapies.

2.5.1.3
Complement

It has been known for many years that C5a is a stimulus for in vitro mast cell histamine release, but it has only been in the last decade that the importance of complement as a co-factor for mast cell histamine release by functional autoantibodies has been recognised [35]. Purification of IgG subclasses from chronic urticaria sera showed functional autoantibodies in IgG1 and IgG3 and occasionally IgG4 but not IgG2 [36]. Since only IgG1 and IgG3 subclasses are capable of fixing complement, this explains why autoantibodies belonging to the IgG2 subclass are not functional, even though they will be detected by immunoassays. It has been proposed that the reason functional autoantibodies cause urticaria but not anaphylaxis is that only mast cells from the skin have the receptor for C5a [25].

2.5.2
Mast Cell Liberators and Pseudoallergens

A number of drugs have been shown to release histamine from mast cells in vitro by a direct (allergen-independent) mechanism including opiates and polymyxin, but it seems uncommon for them to cause urticaria in clinical practice. There were only 124 reports of opiates and 1 of polymyxin causing urticaria out of a total of 9,937 cases of drug-induced urticaria reported spontaneously to the Committee on Safety of Medicines over a 40-year period in the UK [37]. In descending order of frequency of spontaneous reporting were the analgesics and NSAIDs, antibiotics, vaccines, psychiatric medications and cardiovascular medications, but the mechanism for the urticaria was not known and many of these may have been allergic or pseudoallergic (especially the NSAIDs). Although neuropeptides release histamine from mast cells in vitro, there was no evidence of increased substance P levels in the blood of chronic urticaria patients [38] and the contribution of neuropeptides to the causation of urticaria is unknown.

2.6
Tests for Autoimmune Urticaria

2.6.1
Laboratory Assays

Functional assays for autoantibodies still rely primarily on the use of selected healthy donor basophils, with or without the use of IL-3 as a priming agent. Basophils of some healthy donors remain unresponsive whatever the conditions of incubation. A recent contribution to understanding the hyporesponsiveness shown by basophils of some chronic urticaria patients to anti-IgE stimulation has been the finding of increased expression of Src-homology 2-containing inositol phosphates (SHIPs) that appears to be independent of the presence or absence of functional autoantibodies [39]. Basophils of chronic urticaria patients are hyper-responsive to heterologous urticaria sera even from healthy controls but the reason for this is still uncertain [40]. Circulating basophil numbers are reduced, particularly in patients with functional autoantibodies [41, 42]. Unfortunately, they were too low to be measured accurately by the basophil channel of an automated five part differential analyser [41] for use as a potential marker of autoimmune urticaria in routine clinical practice. However, measurement of total blood cellular histamine corresponds closely with blood basophil numbers counted manually [42] and could potentially be used as a surrogate marker. Increased expression of the activation marker CD63 on basophils of chronic urticaria patients on flow cytometry has been demonstrated in vivo but did not appear to be a useful marker of histamine-releasing activity or immunoreactivity to FcεRIα in a small series of patients [43]. However, CD203c expression on healthy donor basophils incubated with chronic urticaria sera was upregulated and correlated with both basophil histamine release and the size of the autologous serum skin test [44]. A correlation with histamine release in vitro was also shown with atopic donor basophils but not non-atopic donors with CD63 expression after incubation with chronic urticaria sera [45].

2.6.2 The Autologous Serum Skin Test

The most widely used clinical test for histamine releasing factors in blood is the autologous serum skin test [46] but it has been criticised for having only moderate specificity and sensitivity for in vitro basophil histamine release in chronic urticaria [4, 5]. It was not abolished by IgG depletion and heat decomplementation [47]. Intradermal skin testing with autologous citrated plasma gave a higher proportion of positive results than autologous plasma and many ASST-negative patients gave a positive APST result [16]. Patients with chronic urticaria and thyroid autoimmunity were more likely to have a positive ASST than those without; the ASST remained positive in the majority of patients with thyroid autoantibodies after clinical remission of their urticaria [48]. The autologous serum skin test remains, nevertheless, a relatively safe and simple test to perform, provides a convincing demonstration for patients that their urticaria has an endogenous cause if positive and may be a useful predictive test for the detection of functional autoantibodies, provided the results are interpreted with caution. It is possible that, in the future, combining information from ASSTs, total blood cellular histamine and activation marker expression on flow cytometry will increase the predictive value for functional autoantibodies in patients with urticaria for clinicians without access to basophil or mast cell histamine release assays.

2.7 A Concept Model for Understanding Chronic Urticaria

A useful way of looking at urticaria from a clinical perspective is to assume that in healthy condition, each of us has an arbitrary threshold for urticaria that is too high to develop

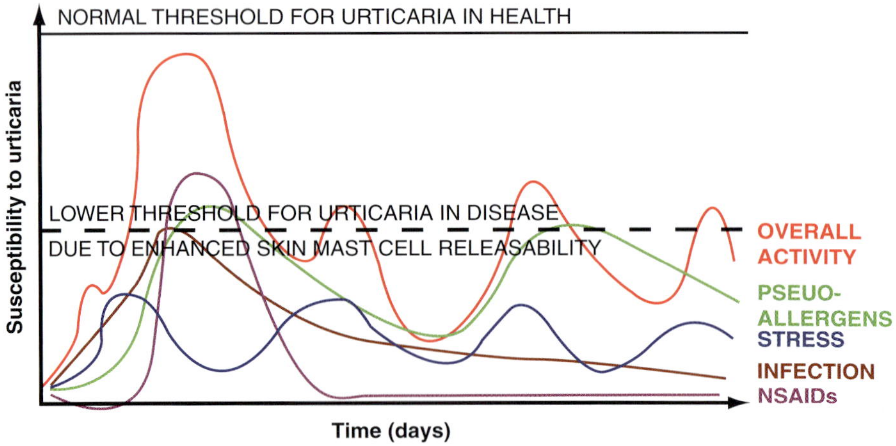

Fig. 2.5 Multifactorial model of chronic ordinary urticaria pathogenesis: the threshold for urticaria is lower in urticaria than in health due to enhanced mast cell releasability. This may be due to functional autoantibodies, or other unknown intrinsic factors. Exposure to external aggravating factors, such as dietary pseudoallergens, stress, acute viral infections or NSAIDs increases the risk of urticaria by enhancing the patient's susceptibility to it. Urticaria breaks out when the susceptibility level crosses the disease threshold, which will vary with the stage of the illness. The day-to-day severity of urticaria may be influenced by the frequency, severity and number of aggravating factors a patient is exposed to simultaneously

symptoms, but during disease activity, this normal threshold drops to a level where urticaria can be induced readily by one or more external aggravating factors acting separately or together (Fig. 2.5). In autoimmune urticaria, the threshold is lowered due to functional autoantibodies. In idiopathic and physical urticarias, the threshold is reduced for reasons that currently remain unclear. As the hypothetical threshold rises as a result of treatment or natural remission of the disease, the same external influences that promote local proinflammatory pathways remain below the "tipping point" defined by the threshold and the illness is no longer expressed. This hypothetical model of the disease carries three interesting implications: first, that some individuals may have a genetically low baseline threshold for urticaria; second, that such individuals may expect to have intermittent episodes of urticaria over their lifetimes with exposure to aggravating external influences, such as drugs and infections; and third, that when the disease is active, there will be many adverse aggravating factors that do not cause urticaria in their own right but can nevertheless contribute to the clinical course. By diligent identification and avoidance of factors that are important for an individual, the risk of severe exacerbations is potentially avoidable, overall disease activity can be ameliorated and the need for emergency treatment can be reduced.

Evidence to support this concept is accruing. An increasing number of reports are coming in of polymorphisms of the beta subunit [49] and the alpha promoter region of FcεRI in aspirin-sensitive urticaria [50] and other potentially relevant targets as the search for susceptibility genes widens. A strong association between chronic urticaria and HLA DR4 has been reported in English [51] and Turkish [52] patients, especially those with evidence of histamine-releasing autoantibodies. Associations with other HLA alleles are being recognised. Patients reacting with urticaria to multiple NSAIDS and antibiotics were found to have positive ASSTs [53] between attacks suggesting that they had an innate susceptibility to urticaria as a consequence of a persistently lowered threshold for urticaria as a result of histamine-releasing factors in their blood. The worsening of urticaria after aspirin and dietary pseudoallergens, including certain food additives, is well established. Ultimately, the aim of management should be to identify what makes urticaria worse and raise the bar by treating the cause (where this is possible) and to modify the disease by second and third-line interventions to achieve better control or full remission.

2.8 Clinical Take Home Pearls

- The transient swellings of urticaria do not lead to permanent damage or scarring.
- Lesional skin biopsy should only be undertaken when urticarial vasculitis is suspected, since the pattern of cellular inflammation in urticaria does not distinguish reliably between the different types.
- Antihistamines should be given at full doses for all patients with urticaria, except hereditary angio-oedema. The addition of leukotriene receptor blockers may give additional benefit when the urticaria is due to dietary pseudoallergens, aspirin or functional autoantibodies.

References

1. Zuberbier T, Iffländer J, Semmler C, et al Acute urticaria: clinical aspects and therapeutic responsiveness. Acta Derm Venereol (Stockh). 1996;76:295–7
2. Shinkai K, McCalmont TH, Leslie KS. Cryopyrin-associated periodic syndrome and inflammation. Clin Exp Dermatol. 2007;33:1–9
3. Russell Jones R, Bhogal B, Dash A, et al Urticaria and vasculitis: a continuum of histological and immunopathological changes. Br J Dermatol. 1983;108:695–703
4. Sabroe RA, Grattan CEH, Francis DM, et al The autologous serum skin test: a screening test for autoantibodies in chronic idiopathic urticaria. Br J Dermatol. 1999;140:446–52
5. Sabroe RA, Poon E, Orchard GE, et al Cutaneous inflammatory cell infiltrate in chronic idiopathic urticaria: comparison of patients with and without anti-FcεRI or anti-IgE autoantibodies. J Allergy Clin Immunol. 1999;103:484–93
6. Toppe E, Haas N, Henz B. Neutrophilic urticaria: clinical features, histological changes and possible mechanisms. Br J Dermatol. 1998;138:248–53
7. Ying S, Kikuchi Y, Meng Q, et al TH1/TH2 cytokines and inflammatory cells in skin biopsy specimens from patients with chronic idiopathic urticaria: comparison with the allergen-induced late-phase cutaneous reactions. J Allergy Clin Immunol. 2002;109:694–700
8. Natbony SF, Phillips ME, Elias JM, et al Histologic studies of chronic idiopathic urticaria. J Allergy Clin Immunol. 1983;71:177–83
9. Smith CH, Kepley C, Schwartz LB, et al Mast cell number and phenotype in chronic idiopathic urticaria. J Allergy Clin Immunol. 1995;96:360–4

10. Hoskin SL, Wilson SJ, Sabroe RA, et al Basophil infiltration of weals in chronic idiopathic urticaria. J Allergy Clin Immunol. 2002;109:A229
11. Cohen RW, Rosentreich DL. Discrimination between urticaria-prone and other allergic patients by intradermal skin testing with codeine. J Allergy Clin Immunol. 1986;77:802–7
12. Asero R, Tedeschi A, Lorini M, et al Chronic urticaria: novel clinical and serological aspects. Clin Exp Allergy. 2001;31:1105–10
13. Petersen LJ, Church MK, Stahl Skov P. Histamine is released in the wheal but not the flare following challenge of human skin in vivo: a microdialysis study. Clin Exp Allergy. 1997;27: 284–95
14. Jutel M, Akdis AS. Histamine as an immune modulator in chronic inflammatory responses. Clin Exp Allergy. 2007;37:308–10
15. Chan CL, Jones RL, Lau HYA. Characterisation of prostanoid receptors mediating inhibition of histamine release from anti-IgE-activated peritoneal mast cells. Br J Pharmacol 2000;129: 589–97
16. Asero R, Tedeschi A, Riboldi P, et al Plasma of patients with chronic urticaria shows signs of thrombin generation, and its intradermal injection causes wheal-and-flare reactions much more frequently than autologous serum. J Allergy Clin Immunol. 2006;117:1113–7
17. Grattan CEH, Dawn G, Gibbs S, et al Blood basophil numbers in chronic ordinary urticaria and healthy controls: diurnal variation, influence of loratadine and prednisolone and relationship to disease activity. Clin Exp Allergy. 2003;33:337–41
18. Kasperska-Zajac A, Brzoza Z, Polaniak R, et al Markers of antioxidant defence system and lipid peroxidation in peripheral blood of female patients with chronic idiopathic urticaria. Arch Dermatol Res. 2006;298:499–503
19. Hermes B, Prochazka A-K, Haas N, et al Upregulation of TNF-α and IL-3 expression in lesional and uninvolved skin in different types of urticaria. J Allergy Clin Immunol. 1999;103: 307–14
20. Toubi E, Adir-Shani A, Kessel A, et al Immune aberrations in B and T lymphocytes derived from chronic urticaria patients. J Clin Immunol. 2000;5:371–7
21. Confino-Cohen R, Aharoni D, Goldberg A, et al Evidence for aberrant regulation of the p21Ras pathway in the PBMC of patients with chronic idiopathic urticaria. J Allergy Clin Immunol. 2002;109:349–56
22. Konstantinou G, Grattan CEH. Food contact hypersensitivity syndrome: the mucoal contact urticaria paradigm. Clin Exp Dermatol. 2008;33:383–9
23. Grattan CEH, Francis DM, Hide M, et al Detection of histamine releasing autoantibodies with functional properties of anti-IgE in chronic urticaria. Clin Exp Allergy. 1991;21:695–704
24. Hide M, Francis DM, Grattan CEH, et al Autoantibodies against the high-affinity IgE receptor as a cause of histamine release in chronic urticaria. N Eng J Med. 1993;328:1599–604
25. Fiebiger E, Maurer D, Holub H, et al Serum IgG autoantibodies directed against the α chain of FcεRI: a selective marker and pathogenetic factor for a distinct subset of chronic urticaria patients? J Clin Invest. 1995;96:1606–12
26. Tong LJ, Balakrishnan G, Kochan JP, et al Assessment of autoimmunity in patients with chronic urticaria. J Allergy Clin Immunol. 1997;99:461–5
27. Ferrer M, Kinet J-P, Kaplan AP. Comparative studies of functional and binding assays for IgG anti-FcεRIα (α-subunit) in chronic urticaria. J Allergy Clin Immunol. 1998;101:672–6
28. Zuberbier T, Henz BM, Fiebiger E, et al Anti-FcεRIα serum autoantibodies in different subtypes of urticaria. Allergy 2000;55:951–4
29. Brunetti L, Francavilla R, Miniello VL, et al High prevalence of autoimmune urticaria in children with chronic urticaria. J Allergy Clin Immunol. 2004;114:922–7
30. Puccetti A, Bason C, Simeoni S, et al In chronic idiopathic urticaria autoantibodies against FcεRII/CD23 induce histamine release via eosinophil activation. Clin Exp Allergy. 2005;35:1599–607
31. Sabroe RA, Fiebiger E, Francis DM, et al Classification of anti-FcεRI and anti-IgE autoantibodies in chronic idiopathic urticaria and correlation with disease severity. J Allergy Clin Immunol. 2002;110:492–9

32. Frezzolini A, Provini A, Teofoli P, et al Serum-induced basophil CD63 expression by means of a tricolour flow cytometric method for the in vitro diagnosis of chronic urticaria. Allergy 2006;61:1071–77
33. Fiebiger E, Hammerschmid F, Stingl G, et al Anti-FcεRIα autoantibodies in autoimmune-mediated diseases. J Clin Invest. 1998;101:243–51
34. Horn MP, Gerster T, Ochensberger B, et al Human anti-FcεRIα autoantibodies isolated from healthy donors cross-react with tetatnus toxoid. Eur J Immunol. 1999;29:1139–48
35. Ferrer M, Nakazawa K, Kaplan AP. Complement dependence of histamine release in chronic urticaria. J Allergy Clin Immunol. 1999;104:169–72
36. Soundararajan S, Kikuchi Y, Joseph K, et al Functional assessment of pathocgenic IgG subclasses in chronic autoimmune urticaria. J Allergy Clin Immunol. 2005;115:815–21
37. Tan EKH, Grattan CEH. Drug-induced urticaria. Expert Opin Drug Saf. 2004;3:471–84
38. Tedeschi A, Lorini M, Asero R. No evidence of increased serum substance P in chronic urticaria with and without demonstrable circulating vasoactive factors. Clin Exp Dermatol 2005;30:171–5
39. Vonakis BM, Vasagar K, Gibbons SP, et al Basophil FcεRI histamine release parallels expression of Src-homology 2-containing inositol phospatases in chronic idiopathic urticaria. J Allergy Clin Immunol. 2007;119:441–8
40. Luquin E, Kaplan AP, Ferrer M. Increased responsiveness of basophils of patients with chronic urticaria to sera but hypo-responsiveness to other stimuli. Clin Exp Allergy. 2005;35:456–60
41. Grattan CEH, Walpole DA, Francis DM, et al Flow cytometric analysis of basophil numbers in chronic urticaria: basopenia is related to serum histamine releasing activity. Clin Exp Allergy. 1997;27:1417–24
42. Sabroe RA, Francis DM, Barr R, et al Anti-FcεRI autoantibodies and basophil histamine releasability in chronic idiopathic urticaria. J Allergy Clin Immunol. 1998;102:651–8
43. Vasagar K, Vonakis BM, Gober LM, et al Evidence of in vivo basophil activation in chronic idiopathic urticaria. Clin Exp Allergy. 2006;36:770–6
44. Yasnowsky KM, Dreskin SC, Efaw B, et al Chronic urticaria sera increase basophil CD203c expression. J Allergy Clin Immunol. 2006;117:1430–4
45. Szegedi A, Irinyi B, Gal J, et al Significant correlation between the CD63 assay and the histamine release assay in chronic urticaria. Br J Dermatol. 2006;155:67–55
46. Grattan CEH, Wallington TB, Warin RP. A serological mediator in chronic idiopathic urticaria: a clinical, immunological and histological evaluation. Br J Dermatol. 1986;114:583–90
47. Fagiolo U, Kricek F, Ruf C, et al Effects of complement inactivation and IgG depletion on skin reactivity to autologous serum in chronic idiopathic urticaria. J Allergy Clin Immunol. 2000; 106:567–72
48. Fusari A, Colangelo C, Bonifazi F, et al The autologous serum skin test in the follow-up of patients with chronic urticaria. Allergy 2005;60:256–8
49. Choi J-H, Kim S-H, Suh C-H, et al Polymorphisms of high affinity IgE receptor and histamine-related genes inn patients with ASA-induced urticaria/angioedema. J Korean Med Sci 2005;20:367–72
50. Bae J-S, Kim S-H, Ye Y-M, et al Significant association of FcεRIα promoter polymorphisms with aspirin-intolerant chronic urticaria. J Allergy Clin Immunol. 2007;119:1280–1
51. O'Donnell BF, O'Neill CM, Francis DM, et al Human leucocyte antigen class II associations in chronic idiopathic urticaria. Br J Dermatol. 1999;140:853–8
52. Oztas P, Onder M, Gonen S, et al Is there any relationship between human leucocyte antigen class II and chronic urticaria? (chronic urticari and HLA Class II). Yonsei Med J. 2004;45:392–5
53. Asero R, Tedeschi A, Lorini M. Autoreactivity is highly prevalent in patients with multiple intolerances to NSAIDs. Ann Allergy Asthma Immunol. 2002;88:468–72
54. Grattan CEH, O'Donnell BF, Francis DM, et al Randomised double-blind study of cyclosporin in chronic 'idiopathic' urticaria. Br J Dermatol. 2000;143:365–72
55. Raho G, Cassano N, D'Argento V, et al Over-expression of Mn-superoxide dismutase as a marker of oxidative stress in lesional skin of chronic urticaria. Clin Exp Dermatol. 2003;28: 318–20

Classification of Urticaria

3

Torsten Zuberbier

Core Messages

- › Urticaria is primarily mast-cell-induced.
- › Depending on the level in the skin where mast cells degranulate, the clinical signs are superficial (hives) or deep swellings (angio-oedema).
- › Urticaria is a disease entity with many subtypes.
- › The symptom weal can also occur independently of urticaria, e.g. in anaphylaxis.

3.1 Definition

Urticaria is a disease entity that encompasses several distinct subtypes. These subtypes need to be clearly differentiated, as diagnosis and treatment differ greatly. Furthermore, it must be emphasised that urticaria is a disease. Weals and angio-oedema, the clinical symptoms, can also occur independently, e.g. in anaphylaxis.

Urticaria is characterised by the rapid appearance of weals and/or angio-oedema (Figs. 3.1–3.6).

Weals are characterised by:

- A central swelling of variable size, almost always surrounded by a reflex erythema
- Associated itching or sometimes burning sensations
- A fleeting nature, with the skin returning to its normal appearance usually within 1–24 h

T. Zuberbier
Department of Dermatology and Allergy, Allergy Centre Charité, Charité – Universitätsmedizin Berlin, Charitéplatz 1, 10117 Berlin, Germany
e-mail: torsten.zuberbier@charite.de

T. Zuberbier et al. (eds.), *Urticaria and Angioedema*,
DOI: 10.1007/978-3-540-79048-8_3, © Springer Verlag Berlin Heidelberg 2010

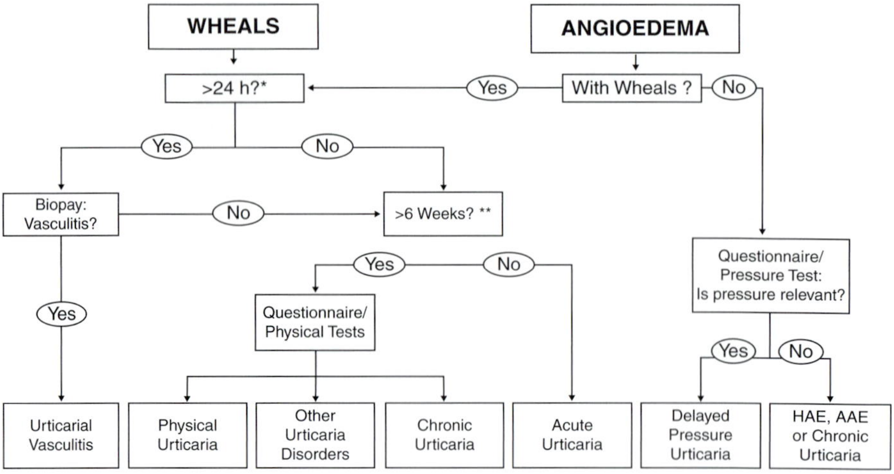

Fig. 3.1 Differential diagnosis of urticarial symptoms. The flow sheets provide recommendations for diagnostic approaches in patients who present with weals or angio-oedema. *HAE* hereditary angio-oedema; *AAE* acquired angio-oedema; *CU* chronic urticaria (ECARF, used with permission)

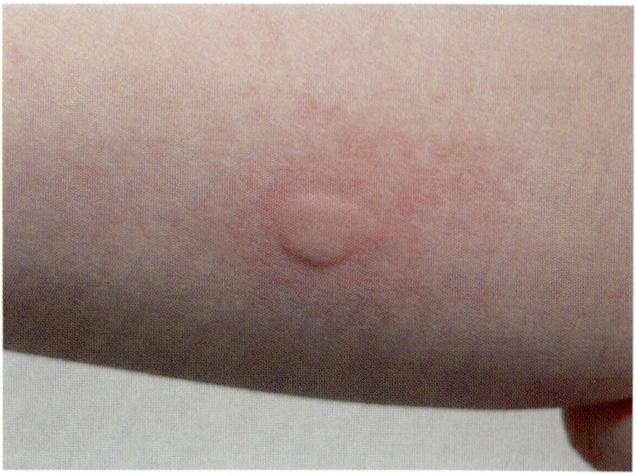

Fig. 3.2 Spontaneous, single wheal in acute urticaria. ©ECARF

Angio-oedema is characterised by:

- Sudden, pronounced swelling of the lower dermis and subcutis
- Occasionally pain rather than itching
- Frequent involvement of mucous membranes
- Resolution, which can take up to 72 h (slower than for weals)

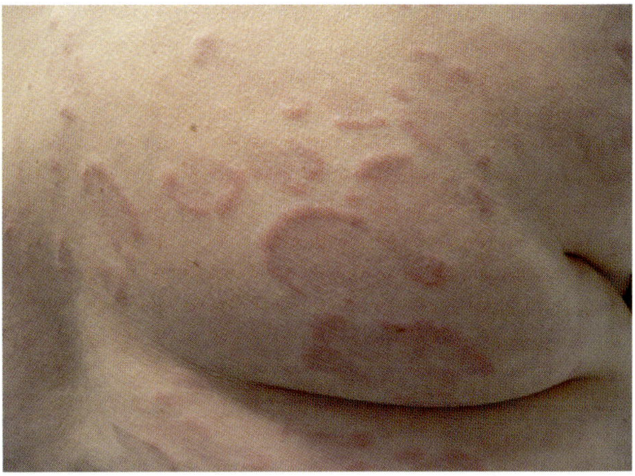

Fig. 3.3 Anular wheals in chronic urticaria. ©ECARF

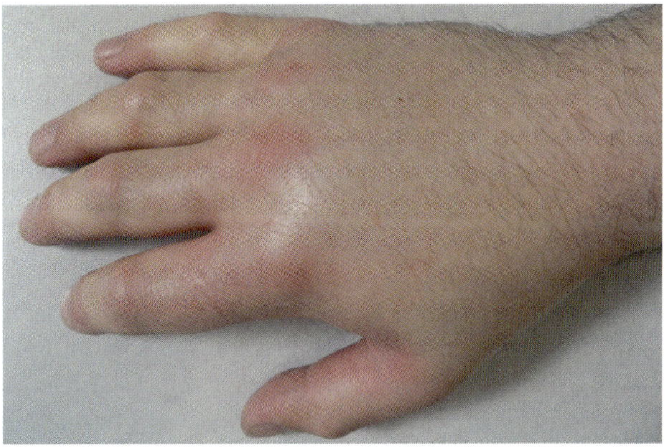

Fig. 3.4 Spontaneous angio-oedema. ©ECARF

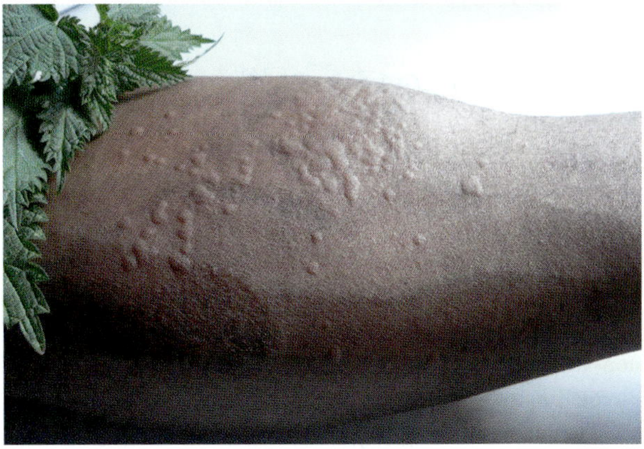

Fig. 3.5 On dark skin erythema is difficult to distinguish, superficial wheals after contact with stinging nettle. ©ECARF

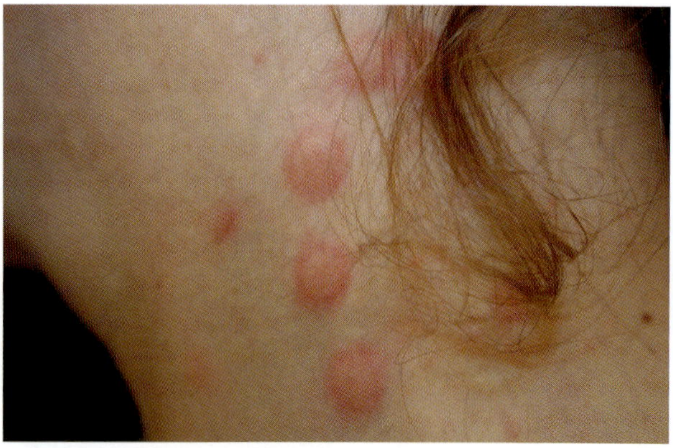

Fig. 3.6 Spontaneous wheals in chronic urticaria resembling an ictus reaction. ©ECARF

3.2 Histology

The classic fleeting weal displays oedema of the upper- and mid-dermis, with dilatation of the post-capillary venules and lymphatic vessels of the upper dermis. Similar changes occur in angio-oedema, primarily in the lower dermis and the subcutis. Weal-affected skin almost always exhibits upregulation of endothelial adhesion molecules and a mixed inflammatory perivascular infiltrate of variable intensity, consisting of neutrophils and/or eosinophils, macrophages, and T-helper lymphocytes [1]. A mild to moderate increase in mast cell numbers has also been observed. In delayed pressure urticaria, the infiltrate is typically located in the mid to lower dermis [2]. In some subtypes of urticaria, upregulation of adhesion molecules [3] and altered cytokine expression can also be seen in uninvolved skin [4].

These findings highlight the complex nature of the pathogenesis of urticaria, which has many features in addition to the release of histamine from dermal mast cells. These changes are also seen in a wide variety of inflammatory reactions and are thus not specific or of diagnostic value.

3.3 Classification of Urticaria on the Basis of Its Symptoms, Duration, Frequency, and Causes

In the last two decades, many advances have been made in identifying the causes of the different types and subtypes of urticaria [5, 6], and the causes that are at the root of the disease's heterogeneity. Among others, chronic infections (such as *Helicobacter pylori*), non-allergic intolerance reactions to foods and autoreactivity functional autoantibodies directed against the IgE receptor have been described [7–11]. However, these different studies show considerable variation in the frequency of the eliciting factor. This may reflect

Table 3.1 Classification of urticaria subtypes (presenting with weals and/or angio-oedema) [12]

Types	Subtypes	Definition
Spontaneous urticaria	Acute spontaneous urticaria	Spontaneous weals and/or angio-oedema <6 weeks
	Chronic spontaneous urticaria	Spontaneous weals and/or angio-oedema >6 weeks
Physical urticaria	Cold contact urticaria	Eliciting factor: cold objects/air/fluids/wind
	Delayed pressure urticaria	Eliciting factor: vertical pressure (weals arising with a 3–12 h latency)
	Heat contact urticaria	Eliciting factor: localised heat
	Solar urticaria	Eliciting factor: UV and/or visible light
	Urticaria factitia/dermographic urticaria	Eliciting factor: mechanical shearing forces (weals arising after 1–5 min)
	Vibratory urticaria/angio-oedema	Eliciting factor: vibratory forces, e.g. pneumatic hammer
Other urticaria types	Aquagenic urticaria	Eliciting factor: water
	Cholinergic urticaria	Elicitation by increase in body core temperature due to physical exercises, spicy food
	Contact urticaria	Elicitation by contact with urticariogenic substance
	Exercise-induced anaphylaxis/urticaria	Eliciting factor: physical exercise

differences in patient selection, underscoring the need for a better classification of patients that will enable the comparison of results from different centres.

Although a number of attempts have been made to classify urticaria subtypes on the basis of underlying mechanisms, the current guidelines [12] do not suggest such a classification, as there is significant overlap between different urticaria subtypes. A classification is therefore suggested to be based on clinical symptoms, duration and frequency.

However, the clinical manifestations of different urticaria subtypes also cover a very wide spectrum. Furthermore, two or more different subtypes of urticaria can coexist in any given patient. The current classification for clinical use according to the guidelines [12] is given in Table 3.1. Some clear inconsistencies are noticeable in this classification; for instance, physical urticarias are chronic conditions, but they are not classified under chronic urticarias because of the special nature of their eliciting physical factors. In typical acute and chronic urticarias, weals arise spontaneously without external physical stimuli.

Urticaria pigmentosa (cutaneous mastocytosis), urticarial vasculitis, familial cold urticaria and non-histaminergic angio-oedema (e.g. hereditary or acquired angio-oedema) are no longer considered subtypes of urticaria, but are listed in Table 3.2 for reference. Chronic urticaria or other subtypes of urticaria are observable in several eponymous syndromes (Table 3.2).

Disease activity must also be taken into account when classifying urticaria. When symptoms arise due to physical triggers, an exact measurement of the intensity of the eliciting factor can be made, e.g. the temperature and duration of application in cold urticaria

Table 3.2 Diseases related to urticaria for historical reasons and syndromes that include urticaria/angio-oedema [12]

Diseases related to urticaria for historical reasons
Urticaria pigmentosa (mastocytosis)
Urticarial vasculitis
Familial cold urticaria (vasculitis)
Non-histaminergic angio-oedema (e.g. HAE)
Syndromes that can be associated with urticaria/angio-oedema
Muckle–Wells syndrome (Urticaria–deafness–amyloidosis), sensorineural deafness, recurrent urticaria (hives), fevers, arthritis
Schnitzler's syndrome monoclonal gammopathy, recurrent fever, arthritis
Gleich's syndrome (episodic angio-oedema with eosinophilia), IgM gammopathy, eosinophilia
Well's syndrome (eosinophilic cellulitis), granulomatous dermatitis with eosinophilia

Table 3.3 Assessment of disease activity in urticaria patients [12]

Score	Weals	Pruritus
0	None	None
1	Mild (<20 weals/24 h)	Mild (present but not annoying or troublesome)
2	Moderate (20–50 weals/24 h)	Moderate (troublesome but does not interfere with normal daily activity or sleep)
3	Intense (>50 weals/24 h or large confluent areas of weals)	Intense (severe pruritus, which is sufficiently troublesome to interfere with normal daily activity or sleep)

Sum of score: 0–6

or pressure, and the duration of application until the appearance of lesions in delayed pressure urticaria. Assessing disease activity is more complex for non-physical acute and chronic urticaria. Several scoring systems have been proposed using scales from 0 to 3 or up to 10 points. The guidelines propose the use of a unified scoring system that would facilitate comparison of study results from different centres. This simple scoring system (Table 3.3) is based on the assessment of key urticaria symptoms (weals and pruritus). It can be used by urticaria patients and their treating physicians to evaluate disease activity.

As urticaria symptoms frequently change in intensity during the course of a day, overall disease activity can most effectively be monitored by having patients record 24-h self-evaluation scores over a period of several days. Additionally, a single time point evaluation and/or sequential physical examinations by the treating physician can help to make the patient's score more objective.

Other issues that have previously not received sufficient attention are inter-patient and within-patient differences in the appearance of weals before and after treatment. In general, larger weals indicate that the disease is more severe and more difficult to treat. The colour of the weals may provide a useful clue to the nature of the disease. Histamine-induced weals are of a light colour and surrounded by a pink erythema, which is caused by the dilatation of cutaneous vessels. Weals of a dark red or violaceous colour may reflect intense vascular damage and leakage in association with weal formation, as found in urticarial vasculitis. Thus, the scoring system should ideally take the size and colour of weals into account, but as these parameters are difficult to quantify, they have not been included in the guidelines.

3.4 Take Home Pearls

- Urticaria can consist of weals and/or angio-oedema.
- More than one subtype of urticaria can coexist in one patient.
- A robust score for assessing disease activity is based on 24 h self-observation of patient's grading symptoms from 0 to 3 for weals and pruritus.

References

1. Haas N, Schadendorf D, Henz BM. Endothelial adhesion molecules in immediate and delayed urticarial whealing reactions. Int Arch Allergy Immunol. 1998;115:210–4
2. Barlow RJ, Ross EL, MacDonald D, Kobza Black A, Greaves MW. Adhesion molecule expression and the inflammatory cell infiltrate in delayed pressure urticaria. Br J Dermatol. 1994;131:341–7
3. Zuberbier T, Schadendorf D, Haas N, Hartmann K, Henz BM. Enhanced P-selectin expression in chronic and dermographic urticaria. Int Arch Allergy Clin Immunol. 1997;114:86–9
4. Hermes B, Prochazka A-K, Haas N, Jurgovsky K, Sticherling M, Henz BM. Upregulation of tumor necrosis α and interleukin-3 expression in lesional and uninvolved skin in different types of urticaria. J Allergy Clin Immunol. 1999;103:307–14
5. Greaves M. Chronic urticaria. J Allergy Clin Immunol. 2000;105:664–72
6. Zuberbier T. Urticaria. Allergy 2003;58:1224–34
7. Juhlin L. Recurrent urticaria: clinical investigation of 330 patients. Br J Dermatol. 1981;104:369–81
8. Zuberbier T, Chantraine-Hess S, Hartmann K, Czarnetzki BM. Pseudoallergen-free diet in the treatment of chronic urticaria – a prospective study. Acta Derm Venereol (Stockh). 1995;75:484–7
9. Hide M, Francis DM, Grattan CEH, Hakimi J, Kochan JP, Greaves MW. Autoantibodies against the high-affinity IgE receptor as a cause of histamine release in chronic urticaria. N Engl J Med. 1993;328:1599–604
10. Fiebiger E, Hammerschmid F, Stingl G, Maurer D. Anti-FcεRI-α autoantibodies in autoimmune-mediated disorders. Identification of a structure-function relationship. J Clin Invest. 1998;101:243–51
11. Buhner S, Reese I, Kuehl F, Lochs H, Zuberbier T. Pseudoallergic reactions in chronic urticaria are associated with altered gastroduodenal permeability. Allergy 2004;59:1118–23
12. Zuberbier T, Asero R, Bindslev-Jensen C, Canonica GW, Church MK, Giménez-Arnau AM, Grattan CE, Kapp A, Merk HF, Rogala B, Saini S, Sánchez-Borges M, Schmid-Grendelmeier P, Schünemann H, Staubach P, Vena GA, Wedi B, Maurer M. EAACI/GA^{2}LEN/EDF/WAO guideline: definition, classification and diagnosis of urticaria. Allergy 2009;64:1417–26

Impact of Urticaria: QOL and Performance

4

Ilaria Baiardini, Fulvio Braido, and Giorgio Walter Canonica

Core Messages

- HRQL is now a fundamental parameter for a global assessment of patients suffering from chronic diseases and it has become a widely accepted outcome in clinical care and research. In addition, HRQL plays an increasing role in the European regulatory documents of pharmaceutical products.
- Because of its clinical characteristics, Chronic Urticaria deeply interferes with physical and emotional well-being, social relationships and daily-life activities.
- As it was recently underlined by the guidelines for CU management, research has only recently explored HRQL in urticaria patients.
- HRQL assessment is now possible by using generic questionnaires or a specific one (Chronic Urticaria Quality of Life Questionnarie – CU-Q_2oL).
- The available studies widely confirm that patients suffering from CU have a reduced HRQL, with considerable limitations in terms of well-being, relationships, daily functioning, sleep, self-image and mood.

A global evaluation of patients must include, together with clinical and instrumental parameters, the assessment of health-related Quality of Life (HRQL). Evaluating the patient's subjective point of view offers a more comprehensive description of the impact of the disease and its therapy on everyday life [1, 2]. This is of particular relevance in patients suffering from chronic diseases, where the primary goal of treatment is to improve their functioning in daily life and to achieve the highest possible level of well-being [3].

In the past, it was frequently assumed that conventional clinical measures of severity provided an extensive insight into describing the impact of the disease. Moreover, the evidence of a weak link between clinical measures and HRQL makes this outcome a

G. W. Canonica (✉)
Department of Internal Medicine, Allergy and Respiratory Diseases Clinic, Genoa University, Genoa, Italy
e-mail: canonica@unige.it

T. Zuberbier et al. (eds.), *Urticaria and Angioedema*,
DOI: 10.1007/978-3-540-79048-8_4, © Springer Verlag Berlin Heidelberg 2010

necessary instrument in the disease management. Moreover, HRQL assessment can improve the physician–patient relationship by giving clinicians accurate knowledge of how patients live with their disease.

While health status is defined by physicians, the impact of a disease on HRQL is assessed by the patient himself by means of validated instruments [4]. Two types of tools are used. Generic questionnaires are applicable to all health conditions; therefore, they allow a distinction between patients suffering from different diseases as well as between patients and healthy subjects. Specific questionnaires are restricted to a particular disease or problem: they are more sensitive than generic ones, but do not allow a comparison between different diseases.

Patients with Chronic Urticaria (CU) report a deep impact of their illness on physical and emotional well-being, social relationships and behaviour: because of the bothersome symptoms, the unpredictable course of the disease, the visibility and the treatment-induced restrictions, urticaria is an irritating and frustrating problem from the patients' perspective. As it was recently underlined by the guidelines for CU management, despite these aspects being a common experience for physicians, research has only recently explored HRQL, namely the impact of the disease and treatment from the patient's viewpoint [1].

The available studies widely confirm that patients suffering from CU have a reduced HRQL, with considerable limitations in terms of well-being, relationships, daily functioning, self-image and mood. Both generic questionnaires and speciality-specific tools have been used for the assessment of HRQL in these patients; recently, an HRQL questionnaire specifically addressing CU (CU-Q_2oL) has been validated [5]. It permits the evaluation of all relevant aspects of HRQL for CU patients: pruritus, swelling, impact of life activities, sleep problems, looks and limits.

People with CU report lower HRQL when compared with healthy subjects or with patients having other medical conditions. This was demonstrated, for example, in a study by O'Donnel, which compared HRQL of 134 patients with those of 98 CU patients with ischemic heart disease (IHD), awaiting coronary artery bypass grafting, by means of a generic questionnaire, Notthingam Health Profile (NHP) [6]. Surprisingly, whilst limited mobility and pain were more severe in IHD patients, sleep disturbance was a greater problem for patients with CU. The scores for energy, social isolation and emotional reactions were similar among the two groups. From the patient's viewpoint, CU causes limitations and problems comparable with those experienced by heart disease patients. In daily life, this burden results in several restrictions and reduced performance. The more frequently reported problems due to CU were: choice of clothing (70%), avoiding social events (73%), sexual life impairment (73%), deterioration of work performance (74%). Focusing on sleep, the study results showed that this component is also significantly burdened: 38% of patients referred high sleep disruption and a further 54% had some sleep interferences. Relaxation during the day was a major problem for 50% of patients and 41% reported some difficulty. NHP results confirmed that the burden of sleep disturbance is marked and that it is greater in CU patients when compared with patients having IHD.

HRQL of CU patients was also evaluated with reference to health status (by means of the generic SF-36) and satisfaction (by means of SAT-P) [7]. Compared with the general population, CU patients reported significantly lower scores in all SF-36 domains; satisfaction levels were impaired by sleep (quality and quantity), physical well-being, resistance to stress and moods. Furthermore, when compared with patients having respiratory allergic diseases (perennial rhinitis and intermittent asthma), CU patients reported a greater subjective impact, with a significant reduction in SF-36 scores (physical functioning, role limitations due to physical and emotional problems, bodily pain, general health and mental health) and life satisfaction (sleep, eating behaviour, psychological functioning and work).

Apart from the generic instruments, speciality-specific questionnaires (developed for skin diseases) were also used. These questionnaires allow the investigation of symptoms, troubles and problems caused by dermatological diseases.

Recently, Grob et al. assessed HRQL in cross sections and matched surveys involving patients with CU (466), psoriasis (464) and AD (426) – The VQ-Dermato, a questionnaire developed specifically for skin conditions, was used. After adjustment on the potential confounding factors (age, sex and subjective perception of disease severity), a typical HRQL profile has been reported for each group. CU patients had significantly lower scores than patients with psoriasis and AD in three dimensions: self-perception, social functioning and treatment-induced restrictions. AD patients registered higher scores than patients with psoriasis in daily-life activities and physical discomfort. Mood state was the only category in which all three groups had similar scores. The mean overall VQ-Dermato score was significantly lower ($p < 0.0001$) in CU (36.93 ± 16.19) and in psoriasis (38.88 ± 17.95) than in AD (44.62 ± 18.25) [8].

Staubach et al. [9] administered Skindex-29 to 100 patients with CU. In line with the results of previous studies, when compared with 96 healthy subjects, CU patients registered a significant impact from their condition on all three domains of HRQL evaluated (emotions, physical symptoms and functioning). This occurred regardless of age, gender, duration of the disease and presence/absence of angioedema. Only the presence of psychiatric comorbidities (depression, anxiety or somatoform disorders) had a greater impact on HRQL. The results of this study indicate that for all its clinical characteristics (symptoms, restrictions, impact on physical appearance, psychological reactions), CU constitutes a relevant problem in most patients; therefore, in the therapeutic approach and management of patients with CU, this evidence should be taken into account.

All forms of CU can have a significant impact on HRQL, regardless of a patients' gender or age [10]. However, it has shown much variation within different urticaria subsets: the association of CU and a concurrent physical urticaria caused the greater burden on HRQL, with significant restrictions in work/study, symptoms/feeling and leisure.

Sleep problems associated with CU constitute a troublesome factor that exacerbates the burden of illness, contributing to impairment of the HRQL [11].

The clinical characteristics of pruritus and its effect on daily life were evaluated in a group of 100 patients suffering from chronic idiopathic urticaria [12]. Most patients experienced pruritus at night ($n = 46$) or in the evening ($n = 37$), rather than in the morning ($n = 25$) or at noon ($n = 18$). As a consequence, sleep was disrupted: 64 patients referred being woken up because of their itch, 62 had difficulties in falling asleep, and 13 took sedatives. In addition, 42 patients were more agitated due to the pruritus and 43 reported lack of concentration.

In conclusion, CU has significant implications for the patient's life, which cannot be neglected. The future HRQL research regarding patients' reported outcomes (HRQL, satisfaction, sleep) may provide data for an optimal management of CU patients.

4.1 Take Home Pearls

- Available data show that CU constitutes a major problem for suffers, with a considerable impact on physical dimension, behaviours, emotions and social life.
- HRQL assessment, by means of validated tools, permits capturing the patient's perspective.
- The international guidelines consider HRQoL a relevant issue for the search of healthcare intervention and the choice of appropriate treatment in patients with urticaria.

References

1. Schipper H, Clinch J, Olweny CLM. Quality of life studies: definitions and conceptual issues. In: Spilker B, editor. Quality of life and pharmacoeconomics in cinical trials. Philadelphia: Lippincot-Raven; 1990. p. 11–23
2. Guyatt GH, Naylor CD, Juniper E, Heyland DK, Jaeschke R, Cook DJ. Users' guides to the medical literature. XII – How to use articles about health-related quality of life. JAMA 1997;277:1232–7
3. Gerth van Wijk R. Allergy: a global problem. Quality of life. Allergy 2002;57:1097–110
4. Guyatt GH, Feeny DH, Patrick DL. Measuring health-related quality of life. Ann Intern Med. 1993;118:622–9
5. Baiardini I, Pasquali M, Braido F, et al A new tool to evaluate the impact of chronic urticaria on Quality of Life: Chronic Urticaria Quality of Life Questionnaire (CU-Q_2oL). Allergy 2005;60:1073–8
6. O'Donnel BF, Lawlor F, Simpson J, et al The impact of chronic urticaria on the quality of life. Br J Dermatol 1997;136:197–201
7. Baiardini I, Giardini A, Pasquali M, et al Quality of life and patients' satisfaction in chronic urticaria and respiratory allergy. Allergy 2003;58:621–3
8. Grob JJ, Revuz J, Ortonne JP, et al Comparative study of the impact of chronic urticaria, psoriasis and atopic dermatitis on the quality of life. Br J Dermatol. 2005;152:289–95
9. Staubach P, Eckhardt-Henn A, Dechene M, et al Quality of life in patients with chronic urticaria is differentially impaired and determined by psychiatric comorbidity. Br J Dermatol. 2006;154:294–8
10. Poon E, Seed PT, Greaves MW, et al The extent and nature of disability in different urticarial conditions. Br J Dermatol. 1999;140:667–71
11. Baiardini I, Braido F, Cauglia S, Canonica GW. Sleep disturbances in allergic diseases. Allergy 2006;661:1259–67
12. Yosipovitch G, Ansari N, Goon A, Chan YH, Goh CL. Clinical characteristics of pruritus in chronic idiopathic urticaria. Br J Dermatol. 2002;147:32–6

5.1 Acute Urticaria

Torsten Zuberbier

Core Messages

- Acute urticaria is a frequent disease with spontaneous appearance of weals or angio-oedema.
- The lifetime prevalence is estimated to be around 15–20%
- The majority of cases are of short limited duration
- Most common causes are viral infections of the upper airways and drugs, especially NSAID

5.1.1 Definition

Acute urticaria is defined by a spontaneous appearance of weals, possibly accompanied by angio-oedema, which last no more than 6 weeks [1]. Acute urticaria must be distinguished from acute attacks of physical urticaria, special types of urticaria or other diseases related to urticaria, e.g., urticaria pigmentosa, where wealing may also occur. This is of special importance since the term acute urticaria implies a disease which is clearly distinguished from the short occurrence of weals for less than a few hours as a symptom of other diseases or anaphylactic reactions. According to the consensus of the German Dermatological Society, a short appearance of weals in a patient with anaphylaxis would be called an urticarial reaction, but not urticaria [2]. This distinction is highly relevant for the interpretation of data regarding the epidemiology and causes of acute urticaria.

T. Zuberbier
Department of Dermatology and Allergy, Allergy Centre Charité, Charité – Universitätsmedizin Berlin, Charitéplatz 1, 10117 Berlin, Germany
e-mail: torsten.zuberbier@charite.de

T. Zuberbier et al. (eds.), *Urticaria and Angioedema*,
DOI: 10.1007/978-3-540-79048-8_5.1, © Springer Verlag Berlin Heidelberg 2010

5.1.2 Epidemiology

According to older literature, lifetime prevalence of acute urticaria, based on questionnaires, ranges from 12 to 15% [3, 4] or even 23.5% [5]. In a prospective study from the Charité [for a doctoral thesis [6], a summary of the data has been published in English [7]], in a rural area of Brandenburg, a 1-year incidence of 0.154% was found, which equals a life-time prevalence of 11.56% based on a life expectancy of 75 years [7]. These data can be considered reliable with regard to the accuracy of the urticaria diagnosis, since all patients were seen by the same dermatologist while still exhibiting symptoms. This was possible because only one dermatologist was working in the area of investigation and all doctors had been asked to refer all patients to him. However, there is no way of estimating the number of patients who believed their possibly mild symptoms to be of minor importance and who did not get in contact with any physician, which is well conceivable in a rural area with a disease that is mostly self-remitting. Thus, the true life-time prevalence for the area may be estimated to be higher, around 15–20%.

In a retrospective representative study performed at the Charité, for the population of Berlin, a 1-year incidence rate of 0.6% was found, pointing to a possible life-time prevalence that is four times higher than that observed in the prospective study in the rural area [8]. However, these data are based on a questionnaire only.

The prevalence of acute urticaria is higher in people with atopic diseases; thus hay fever, allergic asthma or atopic dermatitis were found in 50.2% of patients with acute urticaria in the above cited study of Iffländer [6]. Simons [9] reports on a prospective study in more than 800 12–24-month-old children with atopic dermatitis; in the study group not treated with antihistamines ($n = 396$), acute urticaria occurred in 16.2% over a period of 18 months.

Further epidemiological data revealed a female preponderance of 41–59% [7]; 77% of the patients were younger than 40 years, and 37% were younger than 25 years. The average age was 31.4 years. There was an equal distribution of the prevalence throughout the year [7].

5.1.3 Clinical Aspects

Acute urticaria is mainly characterised by scattered weals (Fig. 5.1.1). The colour is usually light red (88%) and the diameter is usually larger than 1 cm (80%). Weals are accompanied by angio-oedema in less than 5% of patients. In 18% of patients, disease severity is light, with less than 10% of the body area affected; in 42% the disease activity is moderate, with 10–50% of body area affected; in 40% of patients disease activity is severe, with more than 50% of body area affected or systemic symptoms. The reported coexisting systemic symptoms are mild shortness of breath (7.3%), dizziness (2.7%), headache (1.8%), nausea (1.8%) and diarrhoea (0.9%). Full anaphylaxis can occur, but is very rare. In more than 99%, the disease is self-limited and resolves within the first 3 weeks [7].

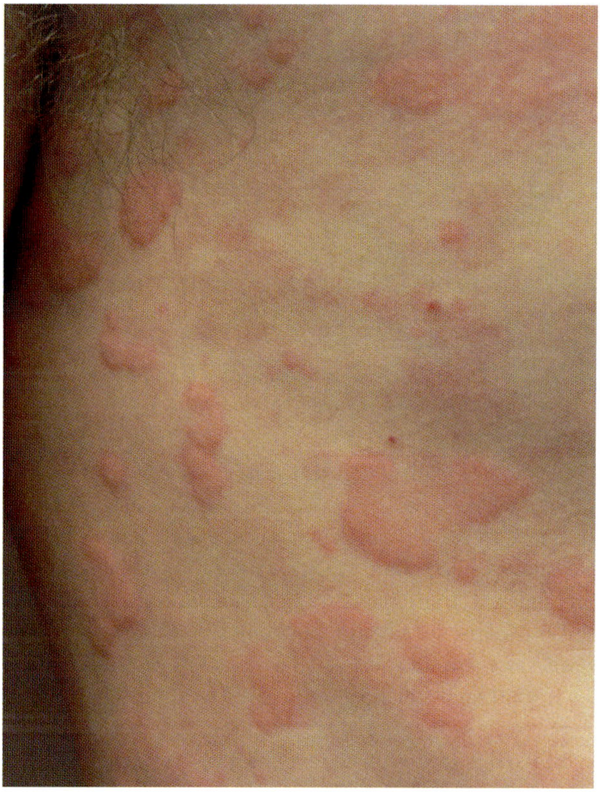

Fig. 5.1.1 Disseminated wheals in acute urticaria. ©ECARF

5.1.4 Aetiology

In the aforementioned own prospective study in acute urticaria, 63% of the patients suspected food to be the cause, since they had consumed some food items in the 2h before the onset of urticaria [7]. However, food was shown to be the causing agent upon thorough investigation in only 1 of 109 patients, which shows that patient history, especially in acute urticaria, may be misleading. However, food is more frequently implicated in children, since Legrain et al. [10] reported food, mainly cow's milk, to be relevant for acute urticaria in 10 of 12 children younger than 6 months of age. In older children with urticaria (6 months to 16 years), Kauppinen et al. [11] observed a 15% prevalence of food intolerance as the eliciting factor for acute urticaria, whereas in an epidemiological study in 50 adult patients by Aoki et al. [12], not a single case of food allergy was found.

Drugs can cause both IgE-mediated and pseudoallergic reactions. While penicillin is the most frequent example of an IgE-mediated drug-induced urticaria, acetyl salicylic acid is the most popular example of a pseudoallergen. The first reaction of urticaria and angio-oedema after acetyl salicylic acid intake was described by Hirschberg in 1902 [12]. In our

Table 5.1.1 Prevalence of upper respiratory infections in acute urticaria

Study	Prevalence (%)
Kauppinen et al. [11]	28
Zuberbier et al. [7]	39.5
Legrain et al. [10]	50
Simons et al. [9]	54.5
Aoki et al. [12]	62

own study, mostly non-steroidal analgesic drugs were responsible for 9.2% of the cases with acute urticaria. These were (acetyl salicyl acid 4×, diclofenac 2×, other NSAID 3×, sulphonizide 1×) [7].

The most frequent cause of acute urticaria appears to be infections, mostly acute viral upper respiratory infections. The rate ranges between 28 and more than 60% of patients (Table. 5.1.1).

A possible explanation for the role of viral infections in acute urticaria is the triggering of mast cells via IgG receptors; however, it is also possible that in addition to the usual IgG response to the viral infection, specific IgE is also being produced under certain conditions. Thus, Grunewald et al. [13] have shown in an experimental model that infection with an influenza A virus can lead to cutaneous anaphylaxis in mice due to the presence of low levels of virus-specific IgE-antibodies. After rechallenge with the antigen, the mice developed virus-specific mast cell degranulation in the skin for more than 48 h.

Regarding the pathophysiology of wealing, similar to other forms of urticaria, the histamine release by mast cells is not the only factor responsible for the symptoms. While the weal itself is clearly histamine-mediated, release of cytokines either by mast cells or by other inflammatory cells, the endothelia, or even keratinocytes may modulate the clinical appearance. While these additional cytokine effects are probably less important in acute urticaria, they are still not negligible in patients with severe acute urticaria. Fujii et al. [14] have shown that in a group of patients with severe acute urticaria who do not respond to antihistamine treatment, elevated levels of circulating IL-6 could be found, while the other mast cell cytokines IL-8 and TNF-α were not increased. The cytokine increase of IL-6, however, was not consistent in all patients, but limited to 9 of 16 individuals. This shows that as in other forms of urticaria, in acute urticaria the pathophysiological reactions are heterogeneous in different patients, which explains the different response to treatment and underlines the requirements for an individual approach.

5.1.5 Natural Course

There are no epidemiological studies available that have monitored the natural course in patients without any treatment. In our own study, the course of the disease was carefully monitored in a follow-up of acute urticaria patients, divided into two treatment groups. The first group received loratadine 10 mg/day until the remission of symptoms, and the second group prednisolone 50 mg/day for 3 days, followed by loratadine 10 mg/day in case

Table 5.1.2 Follow-up of patients with acute urticaria [7]

Cessation of wealing within (days)	Loratadine (10 mg/day) (%)	Prednisolone (50 mg/day for 3 days) (%)
3	65.9	93.8
7	15.9	3.1
14	15.9	1.5
21	2.3	1.5
>21	0	0

After initial treatment with loratadine ($n = 44$) or prednisolone ($n = 65$) for 3 days, all patients were then treated with loratadine (10 mg/day) until remission

symptoms persisted (Table 5.1.2) [7]. None of the patients developed chronic urticaria and the disease can be regarded as mostly self-limited. However, 12% of the 109 patients reported solitary episodes of acute urticaria in the last 6 months to 10 years.

5.1.6 Diagnosis

A thorough examination of patient history is essential and may reveal eliciting factors. However, unless there has been an infection in the last 7 days prior to onset of urticaria or use of drugs (esp. NSAID) on the day of onset, the history is not significant in the majority of cases. According to international consensus, further diagnostic procedures should be limited to cases in which patient history causes suspicion [15]. These may include prick tests (native prick-to-prick) with ingested food as well as provocation tests with drugs at a later time point.

In view of the mostly self-limited disease duration, skin tests or laboratory investigations in patients with suspected reactions to NSAID are not helpful owing to the pseudoallergic nature of these drug reactions, but may be useful for other drugs known to induce IgE-mediated reactions like penicillin. Blood tests for viral antibodies are not helpful, even if viral infections appear to be the most common cause, as they are too unspecific and expansive to warrant their use.

5.1.7 Treatment

According to international consensus, the first-line treatment for acute urticaria is non-sedating H_1-antihistamines, which may be increased in dosage [15]. First generation antihistamines are not recommended to be used due to side effects [15]. The second-line treatment is a short course of corticosteroids; 50 mg/day for 3 days is usually sufficient. According to our own study, an initial short course of prednisolone may reduce the duration of the disease, but does not have any influence on the final outcome, since complete remission occurred in all patients (Table 5.1.2) [7]. Regarding the choice of non-sedating H_1-antihistamines, the general considerations explained in Chap. 6 should be adhered to. Furthermore, in acute urticaria it is important to choose an H_1-antihistamine with a short onset of action at the patient's first visit to guarantee a fast relief of symptoms.

Some of the new H_1-antihistamines are effective as early as 20 min past oral intake and are available as fast-dissolving tablets. Thus, IV emergency treatment is hardly of any benefit, especially since only old sedative H_1-antihistamines are available for parenteral use and require a slow injection over some minutes to avoid side effects like headache. Therefore, IV treatment should be reserved for patients who are at risk for possibly life-threatening systemic reactions or angio-oedema of the throat or larynx, which is relatively rare.

In a double-blind study by Watson et al. [16], i.m. treatment with famotidine and diphenhydramine has been compared. Both treatments were found to be effective, which is very interesting, but the study was not placebo-controlled. For practical reasons, i.m. treatment has no advantage when compared with oral treatment. It is more expensive and has a higher risk of side effects. It can therefore not be regarded as first choice treatment.

In summary, the overall approach to patients with acute urticaria should start with a reassurance of the usually anxious patient that this type of urticaria is not dangerous and is self-limited in more than 99%, and that symptomatic relief can be achieved and that a thorough diagnosis is only required in the unlikely case that the symptoms persist even if no obvious cause is found in patient history. In case of a viral infection in the past, a comforting explanation for the patient is that the weals are a sign of an overactive and potent immune system.

5.1.8 Take Home Pearls

In more than 99% of cases, acute urticaria is self-limited.

- Extensive diagnostic procedures are not suggested except that the patient history renders a specific suspicion, e.g., intake of drugs.
- Type I allergy to food is often suspected by patients but rarely the case/course.
- Modern non-sedating H_1 antagonists are the treatment of choice. Dosage can be increased up to fourfold.
- An initial short course of corticosteroids (50 mg prednisolone per day) may shorten the duration.
- First generation antihistamines are not recommended.

References

1. Zuberbier T, Greaves MW, Juhlin L, Kobza-Black A, Maurer D, Stingl G, Henz BM. Definition, classification and routine diagnosis of urticaria – a consensus report. J Invest Dermatol Symp Proc. 2001;6:123–7
2. Zuberbier T, Aberer W, Grabbe J, Hartmann K, Merk H, Ollert M, Rueff F, Wedi B, Wenning J. Diagnostik und Therapie der Urtikaria [DDG-Leitlinie]. JDDG 2003;1:655–64

3. Sheldon JM, Mathews KP, Lovell RG. The vexing urticaria problem. Present concepts of etiology and management. J Allergy. 1954;25:525–60
4. Champion RH, Roberts SOB, Carpenter RG, Roger JH. Urticaria and angioedema: a review of 554 patients. Br J Dermatol. 1969;81:588–97
5. Swinny B. The atopic factor in urticaria. South Med J. 1941;34:855–8
6. Iffländer J. Akute Urtikaria – Ursachen, Verlauf und Therapie. Dissertation (Med. Doct.) Berlin: Humboldt University; 1999
7. Zuberbier T, Iffländer J, Semmler C, Czarnetzki BM. Acute urticaria – clinical aspects and therapeutical responsiveness. Acta Derm Venereol (Stockh). 1996;76:295–7
8. Balke M. Epidemiologie der Urtikaria. Eine prospektive, repräsentative Querschnittsuntersuchung zu Epidemiologie, atopischen Begleiterkrankungen und Lebensqualitätseinschränkung der Urtikaria. Dissertation (Med. Doct.) Berlin: Humboldt University; 2003 (unpublished data)
9. Simons FER. Prevention of acute urticaria in young children with atopic dermatitis. J Allergy Clin Immunol. 2001;107:703–6
10. Legrain V, Taieb A, Sage T, Maleville J. Urticaria in infants: a study in 40 patients. Pediatr Dermatol. 1990;7:101–7
11. Kauppinen K, Juntunen K,l Lanki H. Urticaria in children. Retrospective evaluation and follow-up. Allergy 1984;39:469–72
12. Aoki T, Kojima M, Horiko T. Acute urticaria: history and natural course of 50 patients. J Dermatol. 1994;21:73–7
13. Grunewald S, Hahn C, Wohlleben G, Teufel M, Major T, Moll H, Bröcker EB, Erb KJ. Infection with influenza A virus leads to flu antigen-induced cutaneous anaphylaxis in mice. J Invest Dermatol. 2002;118:645–51
14. Fujii K, Konishi K, Kanno Y, Ohgou N. Acute urticaria with elevated circulating interleukin-6 is resistant to anti-histamine treatment. J Dermatol. 2001;28:248–50
15. Zuberbier T, Asero R, Bindslev-Jensen C, Walter Canonica G, Church MK, Giménez-Arnau AM, Grattan CE, Kapp A, Maurer M, Merk HF, Rogala B, Saini S, Sánchez-Borges M, Schmid-Grendelmeir P, Schünemann H, Staubach P, Vena GA, Wedi B. EAACI/GA²LEN/EDF/WAO guideline: management of urticaria. Allergy. 2009;64:1427–43
16. Watson NT, Weiss EL, Harter PM. Famotidine in the treatment of acute urticaria. Clin Exp Dermatol. 2000;25:186–9

Chronic Urticaria 5.2

Marcus Maurer

Core Messages

- Chronic urticaria is heterogeneous in its course, clinical picture and underlying causes.
- Autoreactivity, infection and food intolerance are the most common causes.
- Treatment should be aimed at curing the condition whenever possible. This requires the identification of the underlying cause.
- Non-sedating H_1-antihistamines are the first-line symptomatic treatment. The goal is to completely prevent urticaria symptoms from reoccurring, which requires updosing of antihistamines or the use of additional or other therapies in many patients.

5.2.1 Definition

Chronic urticaria (CU) is characterised by the rapid and unprompted appearance of weals or angio-oedema. Weals are short-lived superficial skin swellings of variable size that are associated with itching or burning (Fig. 5.2.1). Weals come with flare reactions of the surrounding skin and they resolve spontaneously (usually within several hours). Angio-oedemas are sudden, deeper, pronounced and sometimes painful swellings of the lower dermis and subcutis of longer duration and slower resolution (usually within several days) (Fig. 5.2.2). They frequently involve mucous membranes. In contrast to all other unremitting urticarias, CU symptoms occur spontaneously, i.e., they are usually not inducible by a specific trigger or eliciting factor. Thus chronic urticaria is synonymous with chronic spontaneous urticaria (sometimes also called "chronic ordinary urticaria") the latter terms allow for a clear distinction from inducible forms of urticaria such as physical urticarias and other forms of urticaria (Table 5.2.1). Notably, these inducible forms are also often of long

M. Maurer
Department of Dermatology and Allergy, Allergie-Centrum-Charité/ECARF, Charité - Universitätsmedizin Berlin, Charitéplatz 1, 10117 Berlin, Germany
e-mail: marcus.maurer@charite.de

T. Zuberbier et al. (eds.), *Urticaria and Angioedema*,
DOI: 10.1007/978-3-540-79048-8_5.2, © Springer Verlag Berlin Heidelberg 2010

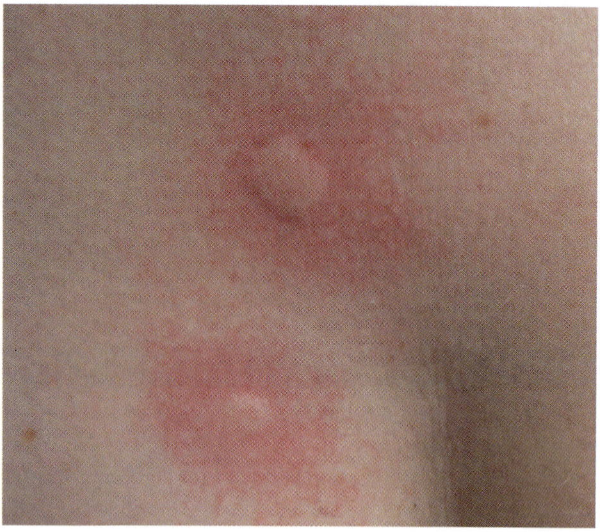

Fig. 5.2.1 Weal-and-flare-type skin reactions in CU patient (ECARF, used with permission)

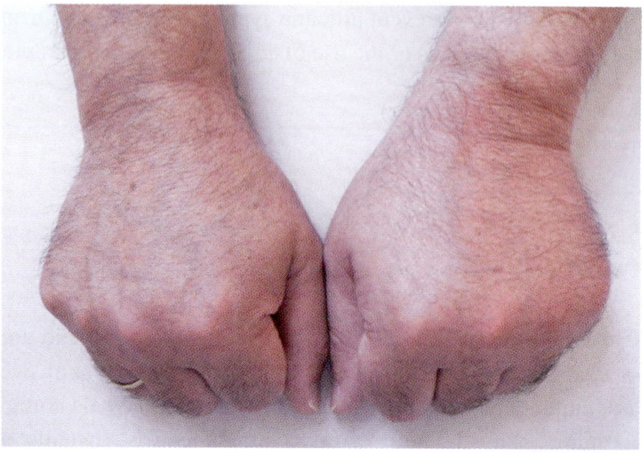

Fig. 5.2.2 Angio-oedema of the left hand in CU patient (ECARF, used with permission)

Table 5.2.1 Classification of urticaria (Adapted from [1])

Spontaneous urticaria		Acute urticaria
		Chronic urticaria
Inducible urticarias	Physical urticarias	Urticaria factitia/symptomatic dermographism
		Cold contact urticaria
		Solar urticaria
		Delayed pressure urticaria
		Heat contact urticaria
		Vibratory urticaria/angio-oedema
	Other urticarias	Cholinergic urticaria
		Exercise-induced anaphylaxis/urticaria
		Contact urticaria
		Aquagenic urticaria

duration and symptoms in CU patients can sometimes be attributed to an inducing factor (stress or physical exercise, for example). Most of the times, however, CU symptoms appear out of the blue, and it is impossible to predict when and why symptoms will appear next.

5.2.2 Clinical Picture

More than 50% of CU patients exhibit both weals and angio-oedemas, whereas about 1 in 3 CU patients show only weals and less than 10% exhibit only angio-oedema [2]. CU symptoms can occur at any time and anywhere on the skin. Most often, however, weals develop during the evening hours favouring the arms and legs [3]. In contrast, angio-oedema is most commonly located in the head region (e.g., eye lids, lips, tongue) as well as in the hands and feet. The appearance of CU skin lesions can be accompanied or preceded by extracutaneous symptoms such as fever, headaches, joint pain, or gastrointestinal symptoms including indigestion and diarrhoea. In about 1 of 10 CU patients, symptoms occur every day (or almost every day) [3], whereas CU in the vast majority of patients is characterised by periods of time in which no symptoms occur for several days to several months. The mean duration of CU is 4 years, ranging from a few months to more than four decades [4], with 50% of CU patients showing spontaneous remission within the first 10 years of disease [5, 6].

5.2.3 Epidemiology

CU is a common condition in all parts of the world. As of yet, very few studies have tried to determine the prevalence and incidence of CU and the results of these studies vary greatly. Most cases of acute urticaria resolve spontaneously within several days or weeks [7, 8] and the risk for acute urticaria patients of developing CU is considered to be low. Different studies report rates of less than 1% to up to 30% [7, 8]. On the basis of older information from the literature, the prevalence of CU is estimated at 1% [9], i.e., five million patients in the EU. More recent studies point towards considerable geographical differences in CU prevalence and markedly higher CU rates (up to 5%) in some regions [10–12]. Women are consistently found to suffer about twice as often from CU as men. The peak age bracket is 20–60 years in both.

5.2.4 Pathogenesis

CU symptoms are brought about by the activation of cutaneous mast cells [13]. Mast cells are large resident skin cells with characteristic metachromatic intracytoplasmic granules containing preformed mediators such as histamine. Mast cells are preferentially localised

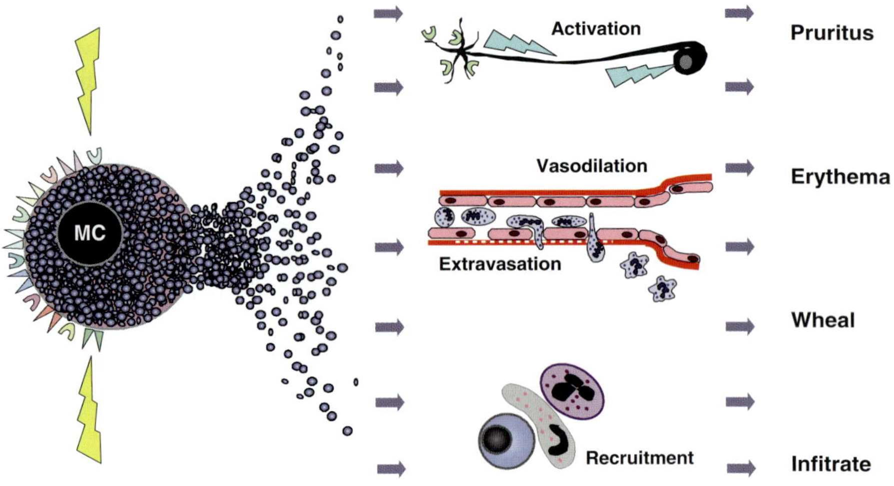

Fig. 5.2.3 Mast cell degranulation and its effects in CU (ECARF, used with permission)

in the vicinity of sensory nerves and small blood vessels of the dermis. Their main physiological role is to provide a first line of defense against pathogens and other environmental dangers [14, 15]. Mast cell activation and the subsequent release of mediators including histamine induce sensory nerve stimulation (pruritus) and vasodilatation (erythema), increased extravasation (oedema) as well as the recruitment of neutrophils and other immune cells (infiltrate) (Fig. 5.2.3). Mast cell activation is a complex process that can be initiated by a large variety and number of receptor–ligand interactions (Fig. 5.2.4).

5.2.5 Causes and Triggers

CU can result from many different causes. The most common causes are (1) autoreactivity, (2) infection, and (3) intolerance. Other causes of CU are less frequent and harder to detect (Table 5.2.2).

5.2.5.1 CU Due to Autoreactivity

About 40% of CU patients express circulating mast cell activating factors [16–18], which appear to be anti-IgE or anti-IgE receptor antibodies in some patients (=autoimmune CU). Up to 80% of patients with CU due to autoreactivity, however, do not express anti-FcεRI or anti-IgE antibodies as detected by Western blot or ELISA [19]. The circulating factor(s) in these patients with "non autoimmune" CU due to autoreactivity remain(s) to be identified and characterised. CU due to autoreactivity is readily detectable by the autogolous serum skin

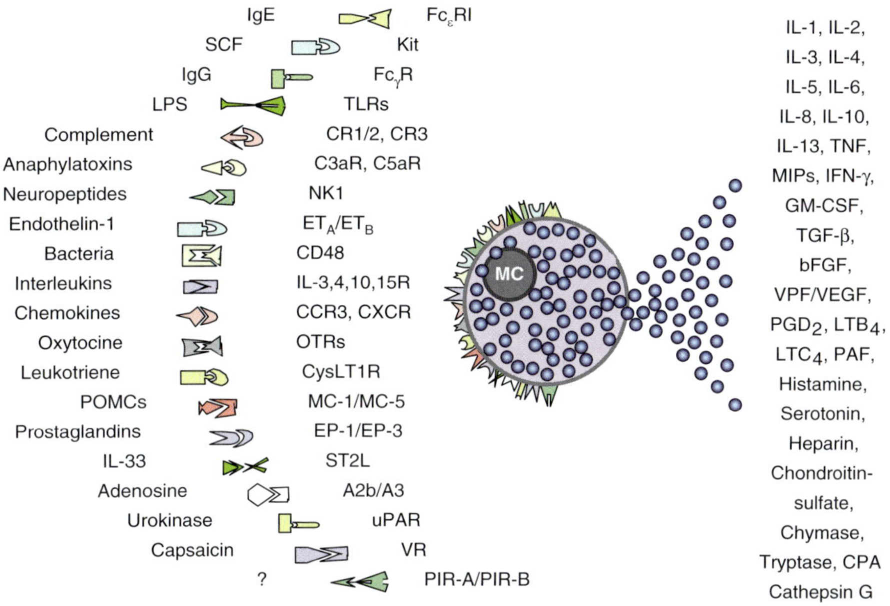

Fig. 5.2.4 Selection of Receptor ligand interactions resulting in mast cell activation (ECARF, used with permission)

Table 5.2.2 Subtybes of chornic urticaria – classification by causes, triggers and mast cell activating mechanisms

Type of chronic urticaria		Underlying cause	Specific trigger	Mast cell activator
Chronic urticaria due to	Autoreactivitiy	Autoreactivity	Not known[a]	Circulating factor
	Infection	Chronic infection	Not known[b]	Not known
	Intolerance	Intolerance	Pseudoallergen ingestion	Not known
	Other cause	Various	Various (usually not known)	Various (usually not known)
	Unidentifiable cause	Not known	Not known	Not known

[a]Potential candidates include autoantibodies against FceRI or IgE

[b]Potential candidates include complement components, immune complexes, pathogen specific IgE, bacterial toxins

test (ASST). The ASST is a sensitive, quick and easy-to-perform "skin provocation test." Patients are injected intracutaneously with 50 μL of autologous serum into the skin of the volar forearm (histamine and sterile saline are used for control injections). In patients with CU due to autoreactivity, this results in a weal-and-flare-type skin reaction. CU due to autoreactivity is characterised by a long duration and high disease activity when compared with other forms of CU. Patients frequently exhibit concomitant autoimmune disorders such as autoimmune thyroiditis [17].

5.2.5.2
CU Due to Infection

Infections that can cause CU include bacterial infections, e.g., of the nasopharynx or by *Helicobacter pylori* of the gastrointestinal tract, parasite infections, e.g., with *Blastocystis hominis,* and viral infections, e.g., hepatitis A and B, [20–22]. Mast cells have been shown in murine models to protect the host from pathogen invasion and from the pathology associated with infection, and mast cells are equipped with multiple surface receptors that function as sensors for bacteria, parasites and viruses. These include toll-like receptors, complement receptors, and Fc receptors. Which of these mechanisms are relevant in mast cell activation in patients with CU due to infection remains to be identified. Also, there are very few controlled trials testing for the role and relevance of chronic infections in CU patients. Generally, CU patients do not exhibit an increased prevalence of infections, and CU due to infection should only be diagnosed in patients who show CU remission upon successful eradication of the infectious pathogen. The most common bacterial infections known to cause CU are *Helicobacter pylori*-gastritis, infections of the upper respiratory tract (e.g., by Group A streptococci), and dental infections. Parasite infections (e.g., by *Toxocara canis*, *Giardia lamblia*, or *Blastocystis hominis*) are a rare cause of CU in Northern European countries, but more frequent in other regions of the world. Intestinal candidosis used to be regarded as a common underlying cause for CU [23], but recent findings do not support this view [24]. Nevertheless, it is recommended that massive candidosis is treated, especially in sensitised patients identified by intracutaneous testing.

5.2.5.3
CU Due to Intolerance

CU patients frequently suspect that their symptoms are brought about by the food they eat. This can be indicative of CU due to intolerance, i.e., non-allergic, dose-dependent and delayed (4–12 h) onset hypersensitivity to food pseudoallergens such as food colorants, preservatives, taste intensifiers and naturally occurring substances, e.g., aromatic compounds, biogenic amines and salicylic acid [25]. CU due to intolerance is diagnosed in patients who show decreased disease activity following a 3–4-week diet low in pseudoallergens and increased disease activity following challenge tests with pseudoallergens. Responder rates vary and range from 50 to 90% following elimination and from 20 to 60% following challenge testing [26].

5.2.5.4
CU Due to Other Causes

Other less frequent causes of CU include type I allergies (less than 1%) and non-infectious chronic inflammatory processes such as gastritis, reflux oesophagitis, inflammation of the bile duct or bile gland, and autoimmune disorders such as systemic lupus erythematosus (SLE).

5.2.5.5 Triggers and Eliciting Factors

Independent of the underlying cause, CU symptoms may be induced or worsened by non-specific triggers. For example, approximately 50% of all CU patients report that physical exertion or stress can reduce the threshold for the onset of their symptoms. Strategies aimed at avoiding or reducing these unspecific triggers can result in less disease activity and a better quality of life.

5.2.6 Diagnostics

Patients should be checked for the underlying cause and relevant triggers of their CU, especially if they exhibit frequently recurring symptoms for more than 1 year and high disease activity. CU activity is best assessed using the "urticaria activity score", a clinical symptom score combining daily values for numbers of weals and intensity of pruritus [27].

The first and most important diagnostic measure in CU patients is to obtain a thorough history including possible eliciting factors and significant aspects of the nature of the urticaria. To this end, all CU patients should be asked the questions provided in Table 5.2.3. This should be followed by a physical examination of the patient including a test for

Table 5.2.3 Chronic urticaria – questions that should be asked

1	When did your urticaria first present? (Life events?)
2	How often do you have weals and how long do they last?
3	When during the day are the weals/the itchiness the worst?
4	What is the usual shape and size of weals and what skin areas are affected?
5	Do you get angio-oedema? How often? Where? For how long?
6	What problems does the occurrence of weals/angio-oedema cause? (e.g., itch/pain/burning?)
7	Does or did anyone in your family also suffer from urticaria (or allergies)?
8	Do you have allergies/other diseases? What do you think is the cause?
9	Can you induce the onset of weals/angio-oedema, e.g., rubbing of the skin?
10	What drugs do you use (NSAIDs, hormones, laxatives, alternative remedies)?
11	Do you see a relationship between weals/angio-oedema onset and the food you eat?
12	Do you smoke/drink alcohol? Do you see a relationship?
13	What type of work do you do? Do you see a relationship?
14	What do you do for fun? Do you see a relationship?
15	Does your urticaria change on the weekend/during holidays or vacation?
16	Do you have surgical implants?
17	Do you react normally to insect stings/bites (e.g., bees, yellow jackets)?
18	What therapies have you tried and what were the results?
19	Does stress trigger weals?
20	Is your quality of life affected by the urticaria? How?
21	In female patients: do you see a relationship with your menstrual cycle?

Table 5.2.4 Basic and advanced diagnostics in chronic urticaria

Step	Diagnostic measure	Goal
Basic	History	Confirm diagnosis, assess QoL
	Physical examination	Exclude major internal condition
	Dermographism	Exclude urticaria factitia/symptomatic dermographism
	Calender/diary	Assess activity and response to therapy
	Differential blood count	Exclude major internal condition
	ESR/CRP	Exclude major internal condition
	Omission of suspected drugs	Rule out drug intolerance
Advanced	Physical skin tests (e.g. pressure, cold, UV, heat) and exercise tests	Verify/rule out inducible urticarias (e.g. physical urticaria)
	Test for autoreactivity (e.g. autologous serum skin test, thyroid: hormones and autoantibodies, ANAs, MCAAs)	Verify/rule out CU due to autoreactivity
	Test for infectious diseases (e.g., stool for *Helicobacter pylori* and parasites, blood for AST and hepatitis)	Verify/rule out CU due to infection
	Test for intolerance to food (e.g., elimination diet for pseudoallergens, provocation with pseudoallergens)	Verify/rule out CU due to intolerance
	Test for chronic inflammatory conditions, type I allergy (e.g., skin prick test, total and specific IgE)	Verify/rule out CU due to other causes

ESR erythrocyte sedimentation rate; *CRP* c-reactive protein; *ANA* antinuclear antibodies; *MCAAs* mast cell-activating antibodies; *UV* ultraviolet; *QoL* quality of life

dermographism for which patients must have discontinued antihistamine and immunosuppressive therapy for at least 2–3 days and 1 week, respectively.

Subsequent diagnostic steps are aimed at the identification of underlying causes and triggers (Table 5.2.4).

5.2.7 Therapy

The overall aim of all CU therapies is to stop urticarial skin reactions and to prevent them from recurring. This can be achieved by the elimination of causes and triggers, by the inhibition of mast cell activation or activators and by blocking mast cell mediators and their proinflammatory effects (Fig. 5.2.5).

5.2.7.1 Removing Underlying Causes, Relevant Triggers and Aggravating Factors

The elimination of underlying causes results in the cure of CU and should be favoured over other therapeutic approaches whenever possible. As of yet, there is no known cure for CU due to autoreactivity. Preliminary reports on the beneficial effects of "desensitisation"

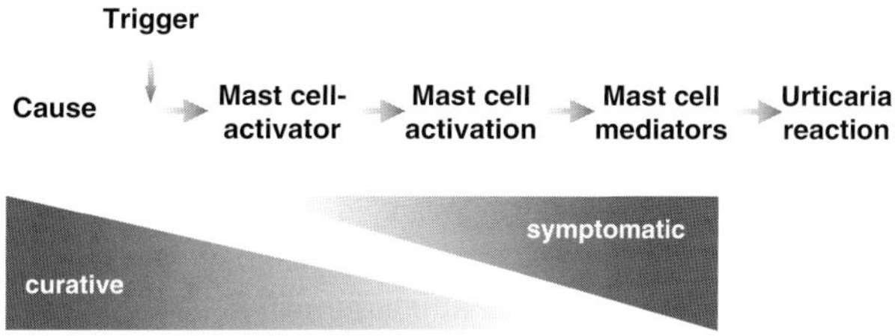

Fig. 5.2.5 Strategies and targets in CU therapy (ECARF, used with permission)

protocols using injections of autologous whole blood or serum require further studies [19, 28]. Potentially relevant infections, e.g., by *Helicobacter pylori*, should be treated and treatment success should be controlled. Responses to antibiotic or antiparasite treatment are known to occur with up to several weeks of delay following eradication therapy. Patients diagnosed with CU due to intolerance are advised to follow a pseudoallergen elimination diet for 3–6 months, after which most patients will tolerate a normal diet.

5.2.7.2 Mast Cell-Targeting Therapies

Mast cells are the key effector cells in the induction of CU symptoms, and inhibitors of mast cell activation or mast cell activators are very effective in the symptomatic treatment of urticaria. Unfortunately, there are only a few drugs available that inhibit mast cell activators or mediator release.

5.2.7.2.1 Inhibitors of Mast Cell Activation

The mast cell inhibitors most widely used in the treatment of urticaria patients are glucocorticoids [29] and cyclosporine [30]. Glucocorticoids, which are effective and safe for the short-term treatment of acute urticaria patients, should not be used in CU patients owing to their side effects of long-term use. Cyclosporine has a moderate, direct effect on mast cell mediator release [31, 32], but cannot be recommended as first-line treatment owing to its safety profile. The principal adverse reactions of cyclosporine therapy are renal dysfunction, hypertension, tremor, hirsutism and gum hyperplasia. PUVA treatment (systemic psoralene plus ultraviolet A irradiation) reportedly reduces the numbers of mast cells in the upper dermis and is thought to inhibit skin mast cell activation [33, 34]. Both UV-A and UV-B treatments have been recommended to be used for CU therapy (in combination with an antihistamine, for up to 3 months) [35, 36]. Sodium cromoglycate (DNCG), which can inhibit mucosal mast cells, does not reduce the activation of human skin mast cells and is not effective in CU treatment [37]. Some modern non-sedating antihistamines have been shown to reduce the release of proinflammatory mediators by mast cells ex vivo and in vitro, but the clinical relevance of these findings remains to be demonstrated. Taken together, mast cell inhibition is not a common approach to treat CU patients because suitable drugs are currently missing. Promising candidates currently under clinical development include raft modulators, tyrosine kinase inhibitors, TLR-ligands and histamine synthesis inhibitors.

5.2.7.2.2
Antagonists of Mast Cell Activators

Antibodies are the only known signals that are relevant for mast cell activation in CU, and these antibodies are only relevant in some CU patients, i.e., anti-IgE or anti-FcεRI (in patients with CU due to autoimmunity) or allergen-specific IgE (in patients with CU due to allergies). As of yet, there is little information on the effects of removing autoantibodies in autoimmune CU patients. Some severely affected patients have been shown to temporarily benefit from plasmapheresis [38, 39]. Also, high-dose immunoglobulin infusions [40] have been reported to be helpful. Because of their high costs, these therapies should be reserved for ASST-positive CU patients in which mast cell activating antibodies have been demonstrated and that are unresponsive to other forms of treatment. Recent findings indicate that the neutralisation of IgE antibodies by omali-zumab injections can effectively reduce urticaria activity [14, 15], but these findings have to be confirmed in future CU studies and randomised controlled trials.

5.2.7.3
Blocking of Mast Cell Mediators

Urticaria symptoms are primarily mediated by mast cell-derived mediators, mainly histamine acting on H_1-receptors located on endothelial cells and nerves. Consequently, H_1-antihistamines are the most important drugs in the symptomatic treatment of CU. As recommended by current guidelines, modern second generation, non-sedating or low-sedating H_1-antihistamines are to be preferred over older sedating H_1-antihistamines whenever possible. Non sedating H_1-antihistamines have been proven to be effective and safe for treating CU patients in numerous randomised controlled trials. They also exert anti-inflammatory effects such as an inhibition of cytokine release from mast cells [41], although it remains unclear whether these effects occur in vivo with standard dosing. There are some studies showing the benefit of a higher dosage of H_1-antihistamines in individual patients [5, 6, 42], but further studies are needed. Because of their good safety profile, second-generation H_1-antihistamines must be considered as first-line symptomatic CU treatment (level of evidence 1^{++}, grade of recommendation A, see Table 5.2.1). In CU patients who do not show complete symptom control even when treated with up to four times the standard daily dose, adding an H_2-antihistamine or leukotriene antagonist is recommended [Zuberbier et al; Allergy 2009; 64:1427–43].

5.2.8
Take Home Pearls

- Patients with long-standing or severe chronic urticaria should be investigated and treated for underlying causes. Autoreactivity, infections and food intolerance are the most common causes.
- Non-sedating H_1-antihistamines are the first-line symptomatic treatment.

References

1. Zuberbier T, Bindslev-Jensen C, Canonica W, Grattan CE, Greaves MW, Henz BM, Kapp A, Kozel MM, Maurer M, Merk HF, Schäfer T, Simon D, Vena GA, Wedi B. EAACI/GA(2)LEN/EDF/WAO guideline: definition, classification and diagnosis of urticaria. Allergy 2009;64:1427–43
2. Juhlin L. Recurrent urticaria: clinical investigation of 330 patients. Br J Dermatol. 1981;104: 369–81
3. Maurer M, Ortonne J-P, Zuberbier T. Chronic urticaria: an internet survey on health behaviors, symptom patterns, and treatment needs in european adult patients. Br J Dermatol. 2009;160:633–41
4. Iffländer J, editor. Akute Urtikaria – Ursachen, Verlauf und Therapie. Dissertation (Med. Doct.). Berlin: Humboldt University; 1999
5. Zuberbier T, Münzberger CH, Haustein U, Trippas E, Mariz SD, Czarnetzki BM. Double-blind crossover study of high dose cetirizine in cholinergic urticaria. Dermatology 1996;193:324–7
6. Zuberbier T, Iffländer J, Semmler C, Czarnetzki BM. Acute urticaria – clinical aspects and therapeutic responsiveness. Acta Derm Venereol. 1996;76:295–7
7. Haas N, Birkle-Berlinger W, Henz BM. Prognosis of acute urticaria in children. Acta Derm Venereol. 2005;85:74–5
8. Zuberbier T. Urticaria. Allergy 2003;58:1224–34
9. Paul E, Greilich KD. Zur Epidemiologie der Urtikariaerkrankungen. Hautarzt 1991;42:366–75
10. Gaig P, Olona M, Munoz Lejarazu D, Caballero MT, Dominguez FJ, Echechipia S, Garcia Abujeta JL, Gonzalo MA, Lleonart R, Martinez Cocera C, Rodriguez A, Ferrer M. Epidemiology of urticaria in Spain. J Invest Allergol Clin Immunol. 2004;14:214–20
11. Ogunbiyi AO, Owoaje E, Ndahi A. Prevalence of skin disorders in school children in Ibadan, Nigeria. Pediatr Dermatol. 2005;22:6–10
12. Vazquez Nava F, Almeida Arvizu VM, Sanchez Nuncio HR, Villanueva Carreto Mde L, Guidos Fogelbach GA. Prevalence and potential triggering factors of chronic urticaria and angioedema in an urban area of northeastern Mexico. Rev Alerg Mex. 2004;51:181–8
13. Maurer M. Allergie vom Soforttyp (Typ I) – Mastzellen und Frühphasenreaktion. In: Saloga J, Klimek L, Buhl R, Mann W, Knop J, editors. Allergologie-Handbuch Grundlagen und klinische Praxis. Stuttgart: Schattauer; 2006. p. 70–81
14. Metz M, Bergmann P, Zuberbier T, Maurer M. Successful treatment of cholinergic urticaria with anti-IgE therapie. Allergy 2008;63:143–250
15. Metz M, Siebenhaar F, Maurer M. Mast cell functions in the innate skin immune system. Immunobiology 2008;213:251–60
16. Maurer M, Metz M, Magerl M, Siebenhaar F, Staubach P. Autoreactive urticaria and autoimmune urticaria. Hautarzt 2004;55:350–6
17. Konstantinou GN, Asero R, Maurer M, Sabroe RA, Schmid-Grendelmeir P. EAACI/GA^{2}LEN task force consensus report: the autologous serum skin test in Urticaria. Allergy 2009;64:1256–68
18. Metz M, Giménez-Arnau A, Borzova E, Grattan CE, Magerl M, Maurer M. Frequency and clinical implications of skin autoreactivity to serum versus plasma in patients with chronic urticaria. J Allergy Clin Immunol 2009;123:705–6
19. Staubach P, Onnen K, Vonend A, Metz M, Siebenhaar F, Tschentscher I, Opper B, Magerl M, Lüdtke R, Kromminga A, Maurer M. Autologous whole blood injections to patients with chronic urticaria and a positive autologous serum skin test: a placebo-controlled trial. Dermatology 2006;212:150–9
20. Cribier B. Urticaria and hepatitis. Clin Rev Allergy Immunol. 2006;30:25–9
21. Federman DG, Kirsner RS, Moriarty JP, Concato J. The effect of antibiotic therapy for patients infected with *Helicobacter pylori* who have chronic urticaria. J Am Acad Dermatol. 2003;49:861–4
22. Barahona RL, Maguina VC, Naquira VC, et al Human blastocystosis: prospective study symptomatology and associated epidemiological factors. Rev Gastroenterol Peru. 2003;23:29–35

23. Champion RH, Roberts SOB, Carpenter RG, Roger JH. Urticaria and angio-edema: a review of 554 patients. Br J Dermatol. 1969;81:588–97
24. Ergon MC, Ílknur T, Yućesoy M, Oźkan S. Candida spp. colonization and serum anticandidal antibody levels in patients with chronic urticaria. Clin Exp Dermatol. 2007;32:740–3
25. Maurer M, Metz M, Magerl M, Siebenhaar F, Staubach P. Relevance of food allergies and intolerance reactions as causes of urticaria. Hautarzt 2003;54:138–43
26. Buhner S, Reese I, Kuehl F, Lochs H, Zuberbier T. Pseudoallergic reactions in chronic urticaria are associated with altered gastroduodenal permeability. Allergy 2004;59:1118–23
27. Młynek A, Zalewska-Janowska A, Martus P, Staubach P, Zuberbier T, Maurer M. How to assess disease activity in patients with chronic urticaria? Allergy 2008;63:777–80
28. Bajaj AK, Saraswat A, Upadhyay A, Damisetty R, Dhar S. Autologous serum therapy in chronic urticaria: old wine in a new bottle. Indian J Dermatol Venereol Leprol. 2008;74:109–13
29. Liu C, Zhou J, Zhang LD, Wang YX, Kang ZM, Chen YZ, Jiang CL. Rapid inhibitory effect of corticosterone on histamine release from rat peritoneal mast cells. Horm Metab Res. 2007;39(4):273–7
30. Harrison CA, Bastan R, Peirce MJ, Munday MR, Peachell PT. Role of calcineurin in the regulation of human lung mast cell and basophil function by cyclosporine and FK506. Br J Pharmacol. 2007;150(4):509–18
31. Stellato C, De Paulis A, Ciccarelli A, Cirillo R, Patella V, Casolaro V, Marone G. Anti-inflammatory effect of cyclosporin A on human skin mast cells. J Invest Dermatol. 1992;98:800–4
32. Grattan CE, O'Donnell BF, Francis DM, Niimi N, Barlow RJ, Seed PT, Kobza Black A, Greaves MW. Randomized double-blind study of cyclosporin in chronic 'idiopathic' urticaria. Br J Dermatol. 2000;143(2):365–72
33. Kolde G, Frosch PJ, Czarnetzki BM. Response of cutaneous mast cells to PUVA in patients with urticaria pigmentosa: histomorphometric, ultrastructural, and biochemical investigations. J Invest Dermatol. 1984;83:175–8
34. Yen A, Gigli I, Barrett KE. Modulation of human cutaneous mast cell responsiveness by a single, low-dose, PUVA treatment. J Allergy Clin Immunol. 1991;88:395–401
35. Hannuksela M, Kokkonen EL. Ultraviolet light therapy in chronic urticaria. Acta Derm Venereol. 1985;65:449–50
36. Olafsson JH, Larko O, Roupe G, Granerus G, Bengtsson U. Treatment of chronic urticaria with PUVA or UVA plus placebo: a double-blind study. Acta Dermatol Res. 1986;278:228–31
37. Thormann J, Laurberg G, Zachariae H. Oral sodium cromoglycate in chronic urticaria. Allergy 1980;35:139–41
38. Grattan CEH, Francis DM, Slater NGP, Barlow RJ, Greaves MW. Plasmapheresis for severe unremitting chronic urticaria. Lancet 1992;339:1078–80
39. Greaves M. Chronic urticaria. J Allergy Clin Immunol. 2000;105:664–672
40. O'Donnell BF, Barr RM, Black AK, Francis DM, Kermani F, Niimi N, Barlow RJ, Winkelmann RK, Greaves MW. Intravenous immunoglobulin in autoimmune chronic urticaria. Br J Dermatol. 1998;138:101–6
41. Lippert U, Möller A, Welker P, Artuc M, Grützkau A, Henz BM. Inhibition of cytokine secretion from human mast cells and basophils by H1- and H2-receptor antagonists. Exp Dermatol. 2000;9:118–24
42. Siebenhaar F, Degener F, Zuberbier T, Martus M. High-dose desloratadine decreases wheal volume and improves cold provocation thresholds compared with standard-dose treatment in patients with acquired cold urticaria: a randomized, placebo-controlled, crossover study. J Allegy Clin Immynol 2009;123:672–9

Dermographic and Delayed Pressure Urticaria

5.3

Frances Lawlor

5.3.1
Symptomatic Dermographism (Dermatographism: Urticaria Factitia)

Core Messages

- Symptomatic dermographism (SD) is a physical urticaria and the most common form of dermographism.
- In SD, waves of itching occur together with an itching wealing response to stroking the skin.
- In SD there is no allergic basis or underlying medical disease.

5.3.1.1
Making the Diagnosis

Symptomatic dermographism (SD) is a condition where unprovoked waves of itching occur and where lightly stroking the skin produces an itching wealing response within minutes.

5.3.1.2
Taking the History

The patient reports severe itching usually out of proportion to any visible wealing and refers to blotches and swellings on the skin. The link between a frictional stimulus to the

F. Lawlor
Dermatology Department, Cutaneous Allergy, St Thomas' Hospital, London SE1 7EH, UK
e-mails: Frances.Lawlor@gstt.nhs.uk, Frances.Lawlor@bartsandthelondon.nhs.uk

T. Zuberbier et al. (eds.), *Urticaria and Angioedema*,
DOI: 10.1007/978-3-540-79048-8_5.3, © Springer Verlag Berlin Heidelberg 2010

skin and the appearance of lesions and itch may not be clear to the patient and it is often necessary to ask direct questions about which areas on the body are most symptomatic and what activities cause an increase in symptoms. In addition, it is helpful to ask about the shape of the lesions. The movement of clothing and jewellery on the skin provokes lesions, and lesions are present where chains worn around the neck or a collar or a strap moves against the skin. There may be lesions around a watch or cuffs and around a belt or near the elasticated tops of socks. For an affected patient, having a shower, particularly a power shower, may cause wealing when the water impinges on the skin, as may towelling dry.

Touching the face unconsciously causes lesions, and rubbing a slightly itchy eye or lip can cause angio-oedema. The lesions occur within minutes of application of the frictional stimulus and disappear within minutes. The longest duration of lesions would be up to 1 h. Patients often report that they are more itchy in the evening.

5.3.1.3 Clinical Findings

The lesions are polymorphic and take the shape of the stimulus applied. They may be linear, square, diamond-shaped or oblong. They are not usually round. As in all urticarias, there may be patchy erythema, papular erythema or weals (lesions with pale compressible centres). All these lesions can occur at the same time. They can change over the course of the consultation. Those patients who are aware of the link between friction on the skin and the lesions often produce lesions especially for consultation, by scratching or rubbing the skin prior to seeing the doctor [1, 2].

5.3.1.4 Confirming the Diagnosis

If the history and clinical appearance are that of SD, the lesions should be reproduced if possible. This can be done by lightly stroking the upper back from above downwards using either a tongue depressor or a dermographometer, which is a device constructed to apply a known amount of pressure. If the patient has SD, he/she will report burning, stinging, itching or other altered sensation within minutes and a weal and flare response will be visible within 5–10 min. It is the combination of itch and weal and flare that confirms the diagnosis.

5.3.1.5 Diagnostic Implications and Treatment

SD is a common physical urticaria, which is also a mechanical urticaria, as it is reliably reproduced by the mechanical stimulus of friction (pressure plus shearing force) on the skin. The condition may occur alone or in combination with another physical urticaria or with chronic idiopathic urticaria (CIU), although it is not considered to be more common in CIU. A diagnosis of SD rules out any allergic basis to the disorder and any associated underlying medical disease by definition. In some patients, the condition improves over 12 months; in others it may be present for 10 years. Patients with mastocytosis are often dermographic on clinically uninvolved skin. Short-lived SD may be produced by scabies, bacterial and fungal infections and reactions to Penicillin and Famotidine. SD may also occur at sites of insect bites, tattoo marks or at the site of intradermal skin testing. Other forms of dermographism include the physiological simple dermographism, in which there is an asymptomatic weal and flare, which occur in 5% of normal people, and very rare forms, for example, red dermographism and cholinergic dermographism, and delayed dermographism which is associated with about 50% of patients with delayed pressure urticaria (DPU).

Treatment should begin by giving an explanation of the condition and regular drug treatment should be started. Histamine is the major mediator released in the condition and SD is responsive to treatment with antihistamines taken regularly. Depending on the severity, it may be difficult to suppress the condition completely. The aim of treatment is to decrease the itching and wealing as much as possible. Some erythema and itch are likely to remain. As the degree of itching is more severe at certain times of the day, it is reasonable to time the ingestion of antihistamine to about 1 h before the itch is at its peak. Often an increase in antihistamine greater than that recommended by the manufacturer is necessary. Giving 12 hourly dosage rather than 24 hourly may help the patient. Second-line treatment, i.e. Montelukast, or third-line treatment, i.e. Cyclosporine, intravenous Immunoglobulin, have not been assessed in SD. Ultraviolet light has been helpful in some patients.

5.3.1.6 Take Home Pearls

- An explanation about the condition is necessary.
- Symptomatic dermographism is responsive to adequate regular treatment with antihistamine.

5.3.2 Delayed Pressure Urticaria

Core Messages

> In delayed pressure urticaria (DPU), there is a delayed response to sustained pressure on the skin.
> Consider DPU in patients with CIU who appear unresponsive to treatment with antihistamines.
> DPU usually occurs in patients who also have CIU.

5.3.2.1
Making the Diagnosis

A sustained pressure stimulus applied to the skin produces a lesion, which usually appears between 30 min and 6 h later and may be present for up to 48 h. Some DPU patients have an identical reaction to friction with frictional stimuli producing similar lesions. This is known as delayed demographism [1, 3].

5.3.2.2
Taking the History

The history is extremely important, particularly as not all patients are aware of the link between a pressure stimulus and the appearance of a lesion. DPU should be considered in all CIU patients unresponsive to treatment with antihistamines. The type of clothing worn and the activities performed have an impact on the lesions produced. The lesions occur frequently in areas where clothing is tight: around the waist area, on the elasticated tops of socks, under straps and under tight shoes. Sitting on hard chairs produces lesions on the buttocks and the backs of the thighs. Driving long distances may produce lesions on the buttocks and across the chest from the seat belt. Lying in bed produces lesions on the head and trunk. Swelling of the hands and feet occurs. The hands swell if carrying bags, using screwdrivers, driving long distances or working using other tools. Feet swell when walking, jogging, running or climbing ladders. Working in the garden can produce hand and foot swelling and knee swelling, if kneeling to do weeding. The lesions are itchy, painful and burning and may last up to 48 h. They disappear to leave normal skin. When they occur near joints, there may be an arthralgia. When the condition is active, there may be tiredness, malaise or rigors.

5.3.2.3
Clinical Features

Lesions of DPU appear deeper than those of ordinary urticaria. Oedematous erythematous plaques and nodules occur. These involve the epidermis, dermis and the deeper subcutaneous tissue. They occur at sites where pressure has been applied to the skin. Occasionally, a bulla may occur. The swelling of the hands and feet is more obvious to the observer on the dorsa of these appendages. A skin biopsy may be helpful. Histopathology shows a more pronounced infiltrate than in other forms of urticaria and can differentiate from urticarial vasculitis. Earlier lesions (less than 5 h) show a preponderance of neutrophils and eosinophils, while later lesions (greater than 12 h) show a preponderance of lymphocytes and eosinophils. The diagnosis can be made after taking a history and clinical examination, but lesions should be reproduced if possible. There are several methods of pressure testing. A positive pressure test consists of the appearance of a palpable lesion at the tested site after 30 min. Most positive responses occur at 6 h. Ryan suspended a 15 lb weight in a crepe bandage over the shoulder, thigh or forearm for 15 min. An apparatus consisting of metal rods, held vertically against the back, has been used by some research workers to reproduce lesions. However, the most convenient and reproducible method of producing a positive pressure test is to use the dermographometer set at a pressure of 9.75×10^5 Pa (99.4 g/mm^2) pressed against the skin at right angles to the back for 70 s. This should be inspected 6 h later.

During an exacerbation, laboratory testing may show an increase in ESR, a neutrophil leucocytosis and an increase in the protease inhibitors alpha 1 antitrypsin and total antitrypsin.

5.3.2.4 Diagnostic Implications and Treatment

DPU is a variable disease with remissions and exacerbations over weeks and months. The response to pressure at any one time is related to the severity of the disease, the amount and duration of pressure applied and the body site involved. The condition may be present for decades in some people. Most patients with DPU also have CIU either concurrently or prior to developing pressure symptoms or later. Other physical urticarias may also be present concurrently. Up to one-third of patients with CIU report exacerbations at sites of pressure. It is not clear whether these patients have mild DPU or whether CIU is exacerbated by pressure in some people. The response to treatment suggests that the latter is true. As previously noted, patients with DPU may also suffer from delayed dermographism.

There is no single effective drug treatment for DPU. Patients need to be given an explanation about the condition and the relationship between pressure and the development of lesions. Patients may be helped by wearing loose clothing. Elasticated belts and soft slightly bigger shoes help. Sports shoes are a good idea. The limitations of treatment should be explained to the patient. While the pressure exacerbation associated with CU normally responds to standard antihistamine treatment, severe DPU tends to be unresponsive to drug treatment. Recommended drug treatment regimes include Cetirizine 10 mg eight hourly, Montelukast 10 mg daily and Loratadine and Montelukast together. One open study suggests that Dapsone is effective and Sulphasalazine 4 g daily was reported effective in two patients. Intravenous Immunoglobulin has induced remission in some. The response to Cyclosporine is variable. Generally, high-dose Prednisolone in a dose of greater than 30 mg daily is useful, but long-term treatment is inadvisable because of the side effects. It would be justifiable to try newer immunomodulatory drugs, e.g. Mycophenolate mofetil or the anti-TNF-α drugs like Etanercept, in patients who are severely affected.

5.3.2.5 Take Home Pearls

- An explanation about the condition is important in delayed pressure urticaria.
- The limitations of the currently available drug treatment should be explained.
- Lifestyle modifications are usually necessary.

References

1. Lawlor E. F. The physical urticarias. In: Leung D YM, Greaves MW, editors. Allergic skin disease. New York: Marcel-Dekker; 2000. p. 195–211
2. Lawlor F, Kobza Black A. Delayed pressure urticaria. Immunol Allergy Clin North Am. 2004; 24:247–58
3. Dice J. P. Physical urticaria. Immunol Allergy Clin North Am. 2004;24:225–46

Heat and Cold Urticaria

5.4

Carsten Bindslev-Jensen

Core Messages

- The patient must be educated on avoiding severe cooling of the skin (e.g., swimming in cold water)
- Some patients develop swellings in oropharynx through intake of cold beverages
- Many cases are seen in combination with spontaneous urticaria
- Severe cases should be equipped with epinephrine
- Antihistamine treatment (high dose) is usually effective in raising the skin threshold level, but should not be used in cases with systemic or severe reactions
- Since prognosis is poor, tolerance induction may be tried

5.4.1 Introduction: The Disease Spectrum

Cold urticaria (cold contact urticaria) is a commonly encountered subtype of physical urticaria characterized by the development of wheal-and-flare type skin reactions or angioedema caused by the release of histamine, leukotrienes, and other proinflammatory mast-cell mediators after exposure of the skin to cold [1–3]. The disease severity ranges from mild urticaria limited to exposed areas in very cold and windy surroundings to generalized urticaria elicited even at room temperature, sometimes accompanied by hypotension and fainting (Table 5.4.1). Several subtypes exist (Table 5.4.2).

Heat urticaria (heat contact urticaria) resembles cold urticaria, but the eliciting stimulus is skin contact with an item with a temperature above the normal skin temperature (e.g., a hot shower) [3, 4].

C. Bindslev-Jensen
Department of Dermatology and Allergy Centre, Odense University Hospital and University of Southern Denmark, 5000 Odense, Denmark
e-mail: carsten.bindslev-jensen@ouh.regionsyddanmark.dk

T. Zuberbier et al. (eds.), *Urticaria and Angioedema*,
DOI: 10.1007/978-3-540-79048-8_5.4, © Springer Verlag Berlin Heidelberg 2010

Table 5.4.1 Classification of cold urticaria severity

Type I	Localized urticaria at site of exposure (most common)
Type II	Generalized urticaria
Type III	Severe, generalized urticaria with hypotension

Table 5.4.2 The family of cold urticarias

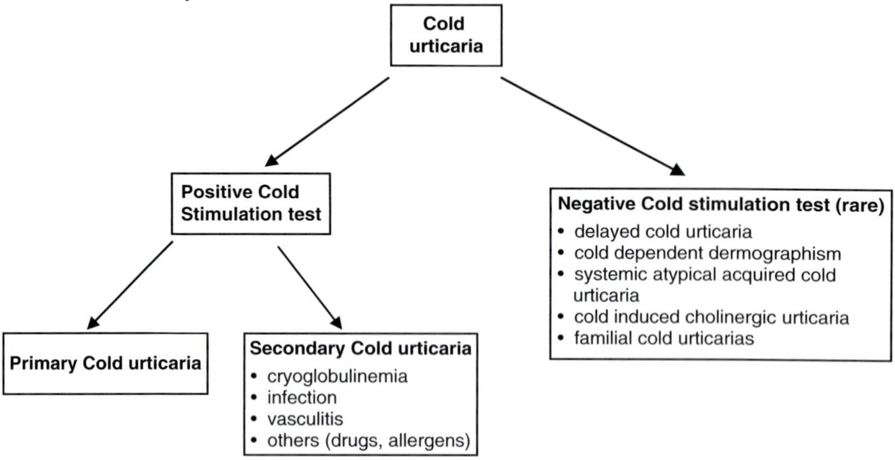

5.4.2 Cold and Heat Urticaria

5.4.2.1 Epidemiology

Heat-induced urticaria is a rare disease with less than 100 cases published [5]. The first report was published in 1924 [6]. Cases in children have been described [7].

In contrast, acquired cold urticaria is one of the most common physical urticarias, ranking third after dermographism and cholinergic urticaria (reviewed in [1]. Prevalence has been estimated to 0.05% in the population [8]. True prevalence studies are, however, lacking and data from German studies indicate that many cases of physical urticarias are mild and, therefore, escape diagnosis by a physician [1, 9]. The highest prevalence of the disease is seen in younger adults, but cases have been reported both in old people and in children [10].

In many cases, cold urticaria coexists with spontaneous urticaria in the patient. Although rare familial cases have been reported, most cases are acquired either without a known underlying cause(s), or – less frequent - secondary to other diseases such as infection (e.g., mononucleosis or bacterial infections, celiac disease, cryoglobulinemia, drugs, allergen-specific immunotherapy, or even malignancies in rare cases [2, 11, 12].

5.4.2.2 Pathogenesis

The central cell in the elicitation of wheals is the mast cell liberating vasoactive mediators on cooling below the threshold [13, 14]. Mediators from neutrophils, eosinophils, and platelets has also been suggested to play a role [15–17]. The mechanism(s) behind the susceptibility of the mast cells to thermal stimuli remains unknown, although presence of IgE antibodies [18] or functional anti-IgE-antibodies [19] has been described. Since 30–40% of patients with cold urticaria have auto-antibodies of IgG or IgM type against IgE or against the high-affinity receptor for IgE [19], and since many secondary cases are seen in connection with infection, a hypothesis of autoimmunity has been put forward.

Little data exist on the pathomechanism(s) behind heat urticaria. In contrast to cholinergic urticaria, where whealing is elicited by an increase in body core temperature, symptoms appear locally by direct contact between a warm item and the skin. An increase in plasma histamine without concomitant increase in serum tryptase after challenge with warm water has been described [10]. A temperature-activated factor in serum has also been described [4].

Histamine is released from the skin mast cells when the skin temperature threshold is exceeded [14], Fig. 5.4.1. Other mediators have been incriminated in the pathogenesis including prostaglandin D2 and platelet-activating factor [20].

Little is known about the pathogenesis of the rare familial disorders, except that Interleukin 1 may be involved in some cases [21].

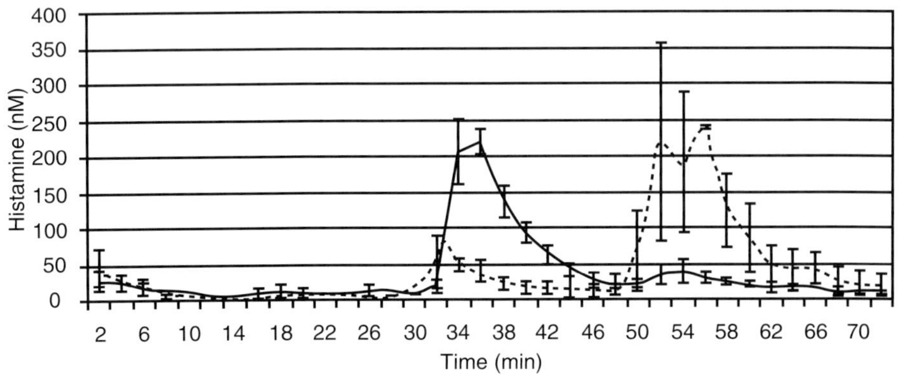

Fig. 5.4.1 Histamine release in three cold urticaria patients before and after passive desensitization. Results are mean ± SEM. Before treatment, all releasable histamine is released on cold challenge, and no residual histamine can be released by codeine. Post treatment, little histamine can be released by cold challenge, but can still be released subsequently with codeine. At $t = 5$ min, an ice cube was placed on the fiber for 5 min duration. At $t = 48$ min, 50 µg of codeine was injected immediately beneath the fiber. From ref. [14]

5.4.2.3 Clinical Features

Symptoms of typical cold (and heat) urticaria can be elicited by exposure to cold (warm) environments, aquatic activities, ingestion of cold (warm) foods and beverages, or handling cold (warm) objects. Severity often depends on the area of the skin involved and on the difference between the temperature of the stimulus applied and the patient's skin temperature threshold. Threshold (i.e., the skin temperature, where mediator release is initiated) varies greatly among patients – the most sensitive patients develop wheals even at room temperature (threshold 20–22°), whereas in others, only application of an ice cube directly on the skin can elicit symptoms. Threshold can be quantified as described later in this chapter.

Most frequently, the major symptoms are immediate development of cutaneous pruritic wheals or angioedema, which may be localized or generalized. The wheals are usually non-pseudopodic and may conform to the shape of the cold stimulus. Following cold exposure to the upper gastrointestinal tract or upper respiratory system, swelling of lips, tongue, pharynx, or larynx may also evolve within minutes. Severe generalized reactions may induce hypotension and syncope (anaphylaxis, Type III, Table 5.4.1). This is especially dangerous if occurring during aquatic activities where the risk of drowning should not be underestimated.

In some cases, whealing can only be elicited in localized areas of the skin; this has been demonstrated in a patient undergoing specific immunotherapy to tree pollen [12].

Other, rare forms of cold urticaria exist [2, 8] and are characterized by negative immediate cold stimulation test (CST) (see later): these include *delayed cold urticaria,* where whealing only takes place hours after stimulation, *cold-dependent dermographism*, where urticarial lesions are elicited by stroking precooled skin, *cold-induced cholinergic urticaria* elicited when exercising in cold environments, *systemic atypical acquired cold urticaria*, where only specific or unique stimuli (e.g., cold wind) can elicit whealing, and very rare hereditary (autosomal-dominant) conditions such as *the familial delayed cold urticaria*, where the members develop delayed reactions resolving with hyperpigmentation and *Familial cold auto-inflammatory syndrome*, characterized by urticaria together with conjunctivitis and fever, eventually also deafness and lymphadenopathy.

5.4.2.4 Confirmation of the Diagnosis

Typical cases of acquired cold (heat) urticaria are easily recognized by patient's case history and can be confirmed by simple CST by placing an ice cube on the skin for 5 min and then observing the developing wheal in the minutes after removal of the stimulus. The CST negative cases (Table 5.4.2) are more difficult to recognize but are much rarer than the CST positive.

Determination of the patient's skin threshold by TempTest® is a new and elegant method to ascertain the severity and impact on quality of life of the patient [14, 22]. This Peltier effect based electronic device (TempTest®; Emo Systems GmbH, Berlin, Germany) allows exposure of the skin to thermal elements with defined temperatures and therefore is ideally

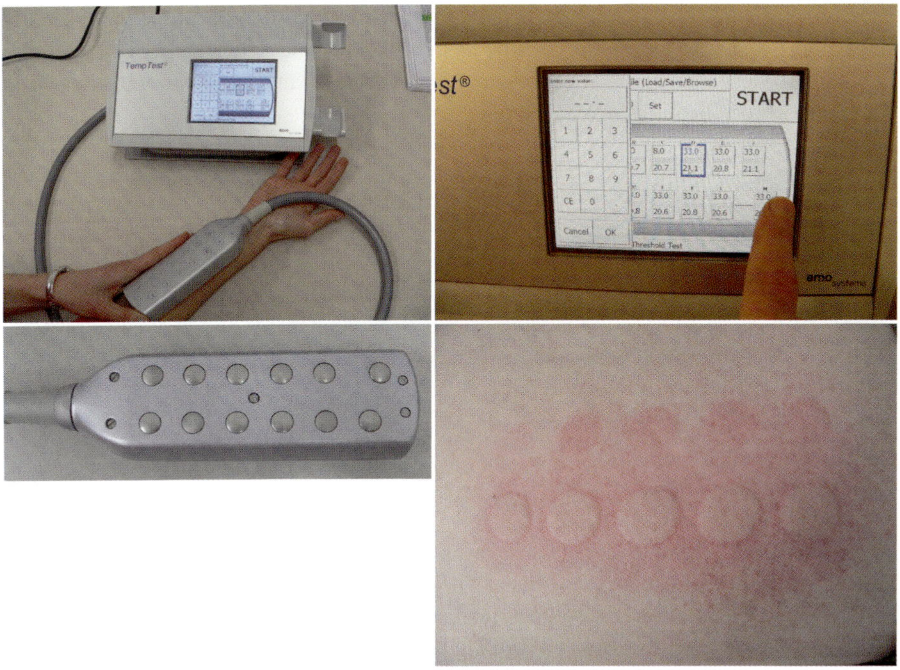

Fig. 5.4.2 Testing for cold urticaira with the Temp Test 3 device to determine the threshold temperature

suited to assess thresholds of both stimulation temperatures and times in patients with cold urticaria (Fig. 5.4.2 – from ref. [8]). Besides determining the threshold levels for whealing, which in most symptomatic cases lies around 16–25° C (resp. above 39° C for patients with heat urticaria), the system can also be used for monitoring treatment response.

Laboratory testing is of limited value in most cases of cold (heat) urticaria [23, 24], and should in cases without symptoms or signs of concomitant disease be limited to evaluation of presence of infection (differential leucocytes count and ESR/CRP). Evaluation of autoimmunity by autologous serum skin test [25] or histamine release from basophils [26] may be helpful in assessing the pathophysiological mechanisms underlying the disease, especially in cases presenting with spontaneous as well as cold urticaria, but are not with our present knowledge associated to the prognosis of the disease.

The cases with negative TempTest are more difficult to diagnose, and field challenge with re-exposure to the actual stimulus described in the patient case history may be necessary.

5.4.2.5 Differential Diagnosis

The diagnosis of primary cold urticaria requires negative outcome in the panel of laboratory tests: ESR, leucocytes, antinuclear antibody (ANA), infectious mononucleosis and syphilis serology, and total complement and cryoglobulin. Cases with positive evidence of underlying disease (cryoglobulinemia, leukocytoclastic vasculitis, hepatitis, mononucleosis, syphilis, celiac disease) are classified as secondary cold urticaria [2, 11]. The rare familial disorders are inherited by autosomal dominant trait, and case history together with the special clinical features may be helpful.

5.4.2.6 Treatment

Avoidance measures, especially for the prevention of shock, are primary in patients with severe reactions. Quality of life is often hampered in the patients and avoidance is rarely efficient as sole therapy. Pharmacologic therapy is therefore often necessary.

5.4.2.6.1 Pharmacological Treatment

Nonsedating antihistamines are in many cases effective in preventing cold-induced whealing and there seems to be a correlation to the increase in threshold temperature measured by TempTest and treatment response. In many cases, however, conventional doses of antihistamines are insufficient in controlling patient's symptoms and in these cases up to four times the recommended dose may be required [27]. It is noteworthy, however, that there are no data concerning a protective effect of antihistamine treatment on systemic reactions with hypotension, so care must be taken to avoid situations where the warning signs (urticarial wheals in the exposed skin, e.g., during aquatic activities) are disguised, thus leaving hypotension and fainting as the first clinical sign of a reaction. Patients with severe reactions should therefore be educated in avoidance procedures and also be equipped with epinephrine for auto-injection.

A course of high-dose penicillin, preferentially administered by intramuscular route, has been reported efficient in a subgroup of patients and may be tried, especially in patients with evidence of chronic infection [3, 28], whereas in a single trial, corticosteroids seem inappropriate [29]. There exist only very limited data on the treatment of heat urticaria [5] – high-dose antihistamine treatment has not been reported, but may very well respond equally to cold urticaria.

Interestingly, especially in the light of the possible autoimmune nature of some cases of cold urticaria, a case of cold urticaria has been successfully treated with anti-IgE (Omalizumab), [30]. A case of familial cold urticaria was successfully treated with anakinra [21].

5.4.2.6.2 Tolerance Induction

This treatment is a cold tolerance induction based on the method of Horton [31] consisting of an induction phase and a maintenance phase. The duration of the induction phase is approximately 5 days where the patient is hospitalized and treatment conducted with resuscitation equipment available. The side effects during treatment are hypotension, headache, and tiredness. First, the patient's hand is exposed to cold water, 15°C, for 5 min causing an urticarial reaction. As the urticarial reaction subsides, the procedure is repeated, usually three times, until further whealing cannot be elicited. By gradually, increasing the exposed skin area, the whole body is finally included. After induction, the patient has to maintain the treatment at home by a 5 min. cold shower every day [14]. Interestingly, as shown in Fig. 5.4.1, in contrast to what was previously believed, treatment efficacy is not due to the depletion of histamine depots from skin mast cells, since codeine stimulation can still liberate histamine from the desensitized patients skin mast cells, whereas desensitization renders the mast cells immune to cold stimulation [14].

5.4.2.7 Prognosis

Cold urticaria seems to be more long lasting than spontaneous urticaria [10, 32, 33] with a mean disease duration exceeding 10 years and with the lowest probability of all types of urticaria of outgrowing the disease [33].

5.4.3 Take Home Pearls

- Heat urticaria is rare but cold urticaria is frequent, especially in areas of cold climates.
- Cold urticaria can be life-threatening in severe cases; in this patient group, emergency kits need to be prescribed.
- Symptoms are related to the degrees of temperature but most importantly also to the wind (wind chill temperature).
- Cold urticaria attacks can be elicited by ingestion of cold drinks and food.
- When patients with cold urticaria undergo surgery, special attention needs to be given, i.e., i.v.-infusions and the metal plate of the table are prewarmed.
- For symptomatic treatment, antihistamines are the first choice; tolerance induction is possible but compliance is often low.

References

1. Kontou-Fili K, Borici-Mazi R, Kapp A, Matjevic LJ, Mitchell FB. Physical urticaria: classification and diagnostic guidelines. Allergy 1997;52:504–13
2. Wanderer A, Hoffmann HM. The spectrum of acquired and familial cold-induced urticaria/urticaria-like syndromes. Immunol Allergy Clin N Am. 2004;24:259–86
3. Zuberbier T, Bindslev-Jensen C, Canonica W, Grattan C, Greaves MW, Henz BM, et al EAACI/GA2LEN/EDF guideline: definition, classification and diagnosis of urticaria. Allergy 2006;61: 316–20

4. Fukunaga A, Shimoura S, Fukunaga M, Ueda M, Nagai H, Bito T, Tsuru K, Ichihashi M, Horikawa T. Localized heat urticaria in a patient is associated with a wealing response to heated autologous serum. Br J Dermatol. 2002;147:994–7
5. Dice JP. Physical urticaria. Immunol Allergy Clin N Am. 2004;24:225–46
6. Duke WW. Urticaria caused specifically by the action of physical agents. JAMA 1924;83:3–9
7. Tomi NS, Schuster C, Bechara F, Hoffmann K, Kranke B. Localized heat urticaria in a child. JEADV 2008;22:384–6
8. Siebenhaar F, Weller K, Mlynek A, Magerl M, Altrichter S, Vieira dos Santos R, Maurer M, Zuberbier T. Acquired cold urticaria: clinical picture and update on diagnosis and treatment. Clin Exp Dermatol. 2007;32:241–5
9. Zuberbier T, Althaus C, Chantress S, et al Prevalence of cholinergic urticaria in young adults. J Am Acad Dermatol. 1994;31:978–81
10. Van der Valk PGM, Moret G, Kiemeney LALM. The natural history of chronic urticaria and angioedema in patients visiting a tertiary referral centre. Br J Dermatol. 2002;46:110–13
11. Delgado MP, Munoz FM, Allue IP, Esteban MM. Cold urticaria and celiac disease. J Invest Allergol Clin Immunol 2008;18:123–5
12. Ducommun J, Morel V, Ribi C, Hauser C. Localized cold-induced urticaria associated with specific immunotherapy for tree pollen allergy. Allergy 2008;63:789–90
13. Andersson T, Wårdell K, Anderson C. Human in vivo cutaneous microdialysis: estimation of histamine release in cold urticaria. Acta Derm Venerol. 1995;75:343–7
14. Petersen LT, Skov PS, Bindslev-Jensen C. Histamine in the skin of patients with cold urticaria – effect of passive desentization. Unpublished results. 2008
15. Soter NA, Wasserman SL, Austen KF. Cold urticaria: release into the circulation of histamine and eosinophil chemotactic factor of anaphylaxis during cold challenge. N Engl J Med. 1976; 294:687–90
16. Wasserman SI, Soter NA, Center DM, Austen KF. Cold urticaria: recognition and characterization of a neutrophil chemotactic factor which appears in serum during experimental cold challenge. J Clin Invest. 1977;60:189–96
17. Grandel KE, Farr RS,Wanderer AA, et al Association of platelet-activating factor with primary acquired cold urticaria. N Engl J Med. 1985;313:405–9
18. Moeller A, Henz BM. Cold urticaria. In: Henz BM, Zuberbier T, Grabbe J, Monroe E, editors. Urticaria: clinical, diagnostic, and therapeutic aspects. Berlin: Springer; 1998
19. Gruber BL, Baeza ML, Marchese MJ, et al Prevalence and functional role of anti-IgE autoantibodies in urticarial syndromes. J Invest Dermatol. 1988;90:213–17
20. Wasserman SI, Ginsberg MH. Release of platelet factor 4 into the blood after cold challenge of patients with cold urticaria. J Allergy Clin Immunol. 1984;74:275–9
21. Maksimovic L, Stirnemann J, Caux F, Ravet N, Rouaghe S, Cuisset L, Letellier E, Grateau G, Morin AS, Fain O. New CIAS1 mutation and anakinra efficacy in overlapping of Muckle–Wells and familial cold autoinflammatory syndromes. Rheumatology 2008;47:309–10
22. Siebenhaar F, Staubach P, Metz M, Magerl M, Jung J, Maurer M. Peltier effect-based temperature challenge – an improved method for diagnosing cold urticaria. J Allergy Clin Immunol. 2004;114:1224–5
23. Kozel MMA, Mekkes JR, Bossuyt PMM, de Bos J. The effectiveness of a history-based diagnostic approach in chronic urticaria and angioedema. Arch Dermatol. 1998;134:1575–80
24. Kozel MMA, Bossuyt PMM, Mekkes JR, de Bos J. Laboratory tests and identified diagnoses in patients with physical and chronic urticaria and angioedema: a systematic review. J Am Aced Dermatol. 2003;48:409–16
25. Sabroe RA,Grattan CEH, Francis DM, Barr RM, Kobza Black A, Greaves MW. The autologous serum skin test: a screening test for autoantibodies in chronic idiopathic urticaria. Br J Dermatol 1999;140:446–52

26. Platzer MH, Grattan CE, Poulsen LK, Skov PS. Validation of basophil histamine release against the autologous serum skin test and outcome of serum-induced basophil histamine release studies in a large population of chronic urticaria patients. Allergy 2005;60:1152–6
27. Magerl M, Schmolke J, Siebenhaar F, Zuberbier T, Metz M, Maurer M. Acquired cold urticaria symptoms can be safely prevented by ebastine. Allergy 2007;62:1465–8
28. Obermayer ME. Treatment of cold urticaria with penicillin. Arch Dermatol. 1963;87:269–70
29. Kobza-Black A, Keahey TM, Eady RAJ, Greaves MW. Dissociation of histamine release and clinical improvement following treatment of acquired cold urticaria by prednisone. Br J Clin Pharmacol. 1981;12:327–31
30. Boyce JA. Successful treatment of cold-induced urticaria/anaphylaxis with anti-IgE. J Allergy Clin Immunol. 2006;117:1415–8
31. Horton BT, Brown GE, Roth GM. Hypersensitiveness to cold with local and systemic manifestations of a histamine like character: its amenability to treatment. JAMA 1936;107:1263–9
32. Kozel MMA, Mekkes JR, Bossuyt PMM, de Bos J. Natural course of physical and chronic urticaria and angioedema in 220 patients. J Am Acad Dermatol. 2001;45:387–91
33. Buss YL, Sticherling M. Cold urticaria; disease course and outcome – an investigation of 85 patients before and after therapy. Br J Dermatol. 2005;153:440–1

Solar Urticaria

5.5

Tatsuya Horikawa,[1,2] Atsushi Fukunaga,[1] and Chikako Nishigori[1]

Core Messages

- Solar urticaria is characterized by wealing in the skin that is exposed to visible light or ultraviolet (UV) light.
- Solar urticaria is usually idiopathic and rarely secondary to porphyrias, drugs, and chemicals.
- Solar urticaria occurs at any age and may be in association with polymorphous light eruption, chronic actinic dermatitis, lymphocytoma cutis, SLE, and other physical urticaria.
- The ranges of action spectra vary among patients, and inhibition or augmentation spectra may exist in certain patients.
- Photoallergens of various molecular sizes have been observed in the patient's sera. Avoiding sun exposure, antihistamines, and irradiation of UV range light may be effective; however, management of solar urticaria is generally difficult.

5.5.1 Clinical Features

Solar uricaria occurs at any age, whereas in many cases it begins between the second and the fourth decades [1–5]. A slight female preponderance has been described. It sometimes occurs in association with polymorphous light eruption, chronic actinic dermatitis, lymphocytoma cutis, SLE, and other physical urticaria, including cold, heat, mechanical, or pressure urticaria [1, 3, 6, 7]. The patient shows well-demarcated wealing at the sun-exposed area of the skin (Fig. 5.5.1). The weals usually develop within 5–10 min of sun

T. Horikawa (✉)
[1]Department of Dermatology, Nishi-Kobe Medical Center, 5-7-1 Kojidai, Nishiku, Kobe 651-2273, Japan
[2]Department of Internal Related Division of Dermatology, Kobe University Graduate School of Medicine, 7-5-1 Kusunoki-cho, Chuo-ku, Kobe 650-0017, Japan
e-mail: thorikaw@med.kobe-u.ac.jp

T. Zuberbier et al. (eds.), *Urticaria and Angioedema*,
DOI: 10.1007/978-3-540-79048-8_5.5,

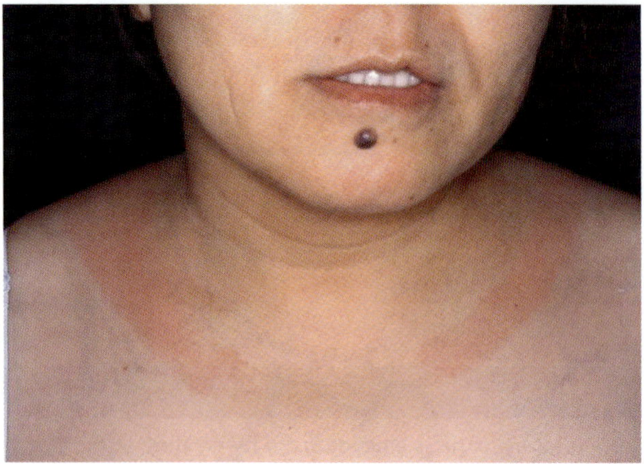

Fig. 5.5.1 A clinical picture of solar urticaria induced by visible light is shown. Note that wealing is not observed in the pigmenting area including face and neck where the skin was frequently exposed to the sunlight (hardening effect) (ECARF, used with permission)

exposure and disappear within a few hours, leaving no particular skin change. Itching or burning sensation is commonly observed at the onset of wealing. Only erythema with itching but without weals may appear when the amount of light exposure is not enough to provoke weals [8]. They may rarely appear several hours after solar irradiation and could persist for more than 5 h [9, 10]. Solar urticaria may occur at fixed skin sites [11, 12]. The covered body area is more sensitive than sun-exposed area such as face and hands. In summer, longer wavelength UV and visible light may penetrate thin clothing, resulting in the development of weals in covered area [2]. Systemic symptoms such as headache, nausea, wheezing, dyspnea, dizziness, and loss of consciousness may occur when a large body area is exposed to sunlight. Bruised skin is more sensitive, probably because photoallergens in serum flow into the skin [13]. The majority of the patients show symptoms perennially, and most of the others during spring to autumn [1, 5, 14]. The proportion of accompanying atopic history varies from 0 to 48% among different studies [1–3, 14].

5.5.2 Pathogenesis

Degranulation of mast cells and subsequent release of chemical mediators including histamine play an important role in the wealing mechanism of solar urticaria, since plasma histamine levels increase after solar provocation [15, 16]. Histopathology at early stage (5 min and 2 h after irradiation) shows the infiltration of neutrophils and a few eosinophils around the dilated vessels in the upper dermis, whereas mononuclear cell infiltrates are dominant 24 h after irradiation [17]. Degranulation of eosinophils may participate in the pathogenesis [18]. Leukocytoclastic vasculitis has been observed in a case with the delayed appearance of weals [9]. Patients develop weals by the exposure to specific wavelengths of light, called action spectra, which variably include the broad or narrow spectra distributing among visible light, UVA, and UVB. It has been shown that patients with action spectrum in short visible range (400–500 nm) have a photoallergen of molecular weight 25–45 kD,

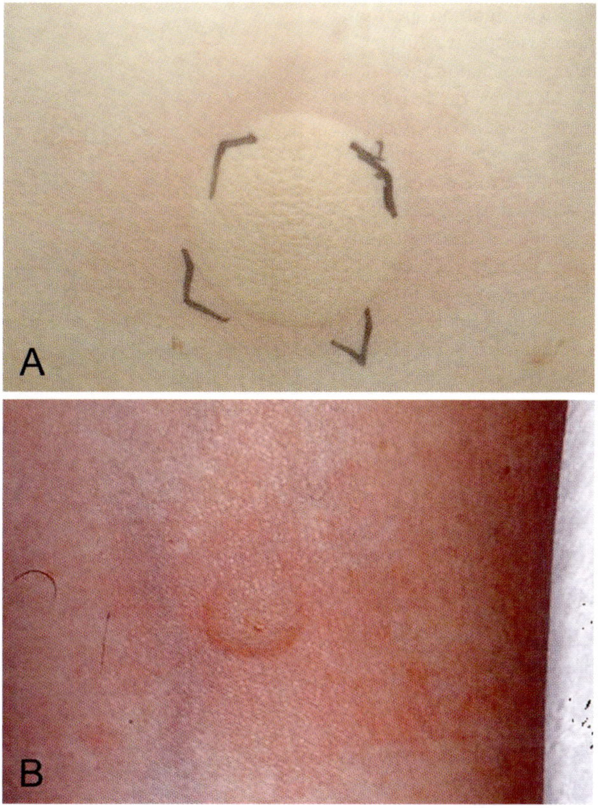

Fig. 5.5.2 (**a**) A weal–flare response is induced by irradiation with a projector lamp, an artificial visible light source. The flare is observed beyond the irradiated area. (**b**) Irradiated autologous serum induced weal–flare response in a solar urticaria patient (ECARF, used with permission)

while those with action spectrum in UVA and short visible light range (330–520 nm) have another photoallergen of molecular weight 300–1,000 kD [19]. Other investigators have described that a case with action spectrum in short visible range had higher molecular weight (over 100 kD) [20]. Photoallergens over 300 kD have been suggested to be the responsible factors in a patient showing action spectrum of UVA and visible light range [21]. Broadband sources such as a xenon lamp, sunlamps, fluorescent black lights, and a projector lamp are useful for the determination of action spectrum when wavelength-specific cutoff filters are combined (Figs. 5.5.2a and 5.5.3a). Phototesting using monochromator reveals more precise action spectra. The majority of the patients in England, Scotland, and Belgium are sensitive to broad range from UV to visible light [1, 7, 14], while those in Italy and Japan are to visible range alone [3, 5]. Action spectrum may vary from time to time in the same patient [22].

Hasei et al. have described that wealing induced by action spectrum is inhibited by the exposure to a longer wavelength light, which is called inhibition spectrum (Fig. 5.5.3b) [23]. This inhibition spectrum suppresses weal–flare response when it is irradiated before, during, and immediately after the irradiation of action spectrum [5, 23–26]. In a series of Japanese patients, 13 of 19 patients had inhibition spectra, of which wavelengths were longer than action spectra in 12 cases [5]. Rarely, an irradiation of longer or shorter

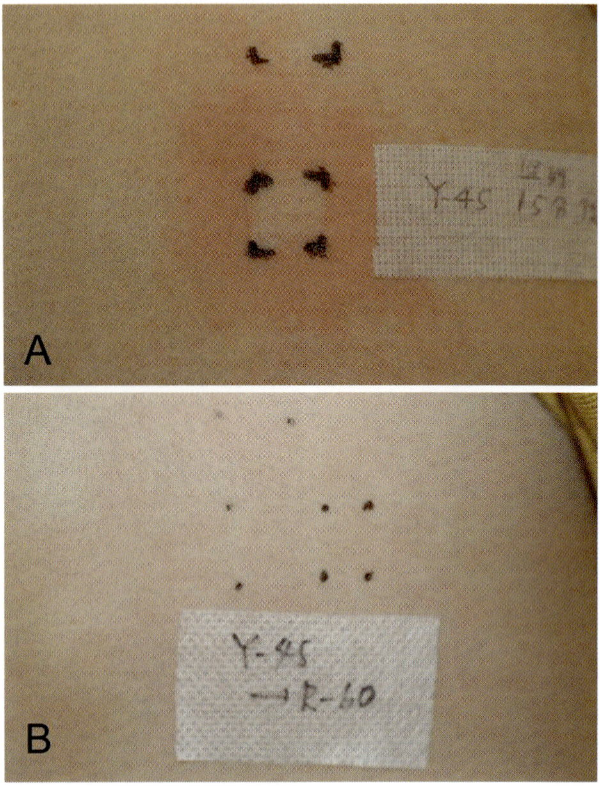

Fig. 5.5.3 Inhibition spectrum suppresses the wealing induced by action spectrum. (**a**) An exposure of visible light at more than 450 nm for 10 min induces wealing 5 min later in a patient. (**b**) Additional exposure of the light at more than 600 nm immediately after the irradiation of more than 450 nm light inhibited wealing in the same patient (ECARF, used with permission)

wavelength light may augment wealing induced by the irradiation of action spectrum [5, 27, 28]. Inhibition and augmentation spectrum may be found in the same individual.

Transfer of patient's serum into a healthy individual and a subsequent irradiation of action spectrum can cause urticaria [19, 29, 30]. IgE is a probable transferable factor in this transfer study [15, 31]. Irradiation of normal skin in a healthy individual and subsequent transfer of patient's serum may induce weals in some cases [32]. It is well known that wealing is frequently provoked when irradiated autologous serum is injected into the patient's skin, suggesting that autologous photoallergens participate in the pathogenesis (Fig. 5.5.2b) [19, 22, 27, 55]. In contrast, the injection of irradiated serum of a normal individual into the patient's skin does not always induce wealing in such patients [33]. In our study, the inhibition spectrum suppressed wealing induced by the dermal injection of photo-activated autologous serum but not of compound 48/80 or histamine [34], implying that inhibition spectrum might affect the intercalation between photoallergen and mast cell.

Leenutaphong et al. proposed two types of solar urticaria: IgE-mediated hypersensitivity to patient-specific photoallergens and that to common photoallergens generally found in healthy individuals [35]. The former reacts to specific photoallergens that are generated only in patients, while the latter respond to nonspecific photoallergens that ubiquitously exist even in normal persons. The responsible photoallergens are not identified so far. Harber classified solar urticaria into six types based on the features of action spectrum and passive transfer test, indicating that it may be a complex disease caused by various causations [29]. Porphyrin is a chromophor for 400 nm wavelength, and could be a causation of solar urticaria. Erythropoietic porphyria and porphyria cutanea tarda may be rarely associated with solar urticaria [36]. In a patient with porphyria cutanea tarda who did not show solar urticaria clinically, experimental light irradiation at 400 nm could induce wealing, which was inhibited by a longer wavelength light [37]. Solar urticaria is possibly caused by drugs including chlorpromazine [38], tetracycline [39], repirinast [40], and progesterone compounds [41]. Contact with chemicals such as tar and pitch could be another causation [42].

5.5.3 Treatment and Prognosis

The management of the symptoms of solar urticaria is rather difficult, because it frequently resists to the treatment. Protection from solar radiation using hat, dark clothing, and a broad-spectrum sunscreen prevents wealing in patients with mild symptoms. It would be, however, difficult to achieve a complete avoidance of the light under the sun in daily life. Sunscreens are effective for the prevention from UV light but not from visible light. Non-sedating H_1 antihistamines, especially at higher doses, weaken the symptoms including wealing and itching, but in many cases fail to prevent the symptoms [2, 4]. Two-thirds of the patients may have at least some benefit by taking H_1 antihistamines, and about one-third of the patients have very good response [1, 3]. Cimetidine, a H_2 antihistamine, has been reported to be effective in a patient, even if H_1 antihistamines are ineffective [43]. Repeated exposure to the sunlight may induce tolerance, although spontaneous hardening occurs in less than 30% [1, 14]. To obtain tolerance, phototherapeutic irradiation of UVA, broadband UVB, or narrowband UVB appears to be useful [44–49]. This hardening effect lasts for a few days as spontaneous tolerance by solar exposure does [2]. Photochemotherapy using 8-methoxypsoralen with UVA irradiation seems to have prolonged effect [50]. Alternative treatments including doxepin [51], cyclosporine [52], intravenous immunoglobulin [53], photopheresis [54], and plasmapheresis [55] have been reported to be effective. Beta-carotene seems to be ineffective [4] and antimalarials may be effective in certain patients [56, 57]. It has been suggested that a combination of these treatments is required for the control of symptoms and the improvement in quality of life [2].

Prognosis of solar urticaria seems to be unclear. The severity of the disease alters in time. Actually, minimal urticarial dose may increase or decrease after a long time follow-up [22]. Some patients become disease-free several years later, although others do not. In a series of 87 patients with solar urticaria, the probability of resolution after diagnosis is 12% at 5 years, 26% at 10 years, and 36% at 15 years [1]. In contrast, it has been reported that 57.5% of patients with solar urticaria were resolved at 5 years in a series of 57 cases [3].

5.5.4 Take Home Pearls

- Sunscreens are effective for the prevention from UV light when the action spectra are within UV range.
- Autologous photoallergens that react with IgE antibodies have been suggested to participate in the pathogenesis.
- Solar urticaria may be induced by chlorpromazine, tetracycline, repirinast, and progesterone compounds.
- Two-thirds of the patients may have at least some benefit by taking H_1 antihistamines, and about a third of the patients have very good response.
- Repeated exposure to the sunlight, UVA, or UVB may induce tolerance in certain patients, and PUVA seems to have prolonged effect.
- Resolution at 5 years varies from 12 to 57.5% according to the different reports.

References

1. Beattie PE, Dawe RS, Ibbotson SH, Ferguson J. Characteristics and prognosis of idiopathic solar urticaria. A cohort of 87 cases. Arch Dermatol. 2003;139:1149–54
2. Horio T. Solar urticaria-idiopathic? Photodermatol Photoimmunol Photomed. 2003;19:147–54
3. Monfrecola G, Masturzo E, Riccardo AM, Balato F, Ayala F, Di Costanzo MP. Solar urticaria: a report on 57 cases. Am J Contact Dermatol. 2000;11:89–94
4. Roelandts R, Ryckaert S. Solar urticaria: the annoying photodermatosis. Int J Dermatol. 1999; 38:411–8
5. Uetsu N, Miyauchi-Hashimoto H, Okamoto H, Horio T. The clinical and photobiological characteristics of solar urticaria in 40 patients. Br J Dermatol. 2000;142:32–8
6. Delorme P, Giroux JM. Solar urticaria as the presenting manifestation of systemic lupus erythematosus. Can Med Assoc J. 1966;95:539–42
7. Frain-Bell W. Solar urticaria. In: Frain-Bell W, editor. Cutaneous photobiology. Oxford: Oxford University Press; 1985. p. 51–5
8. Torinuki W. Two patients with solar urticaria manifesting pruritic erythema. J Dermatol. 1992;19:635–7
9. Armstrong RB, Horan DB, Silvers DN. Leukocyteclastic vasculitits in urticaria induced by ultraviolet irradiation. Arch Dermatol. 1985;121:1145–8
10. Monfrecola G, Nappa P, Pini D. Solar urticaria with delayed onset: a case report. Photodermatology 1988;5:103–4
11. Reinauer S, Leenutaphong V, Holzle E. Fixed solar urticaria. J Am Acad Dermatol. 1993;29:161–5
12. Soter NA, Wasserman SI, Pathak MA, Parish JA, Austen KF. Solar urticaria: release of mast cell mediators in to the circulation after experimental challenge. J Invest Dermatol. 1979;72: 282–300
13. Norris PG, Hawk JLM. Bruising and susceptibility to solar urticaria. Brit J Dermatol. 1991;124:393
14. Ryckaert S, Roelandts R. Solar urticaria: a report of 25 cases and difficulties in phototesting. Arch Dermatol. 1998;134:71–4

15. Hawk JL, Eady RA, Challoner AV, Kobza-Black A, Keahey TM, Greaves MW. Elevated blood histamine levels and mast cell degranulation in solar urticaria. Br J Clin Pharmacol. 1980;9: 183–6
16. Schwarze HP, Marguery MC, Journe F, Loche F, Bazex J. Fixed solar urticaria to visible light successfully treated with fexofenadine. Photodermatol Photoimmunol Photomed. 2001;17: 39–41
17. Norris PG, Murphy GM, Hawk JLM, Winkelmann RK. A histological study of the evolution of solar urticaria. Arch Dermatol. 1988;124:80–3
18. Leiferman KM, Norris PG, Murphy GM, Hawk JLM, Winkelmann RK. Evidence for eosinophil degranulation with deposition of granule major basic protein in solar urticaria. J Am Acad Dermatol. 1989;21:75–80
19. Kojima M, Horiko T, Nakamura Y, Aoki T. Solar urticaria: the relationship of photoallergen and action spectrum. Arch Dermatol. 1986;122:550–5
20. Horio T. Photoallergic urticaria induced by visible light: additional cases and further study. Arch Dermatol. 1978;114:1761–4
21. Miyauchi H, Horio T. Detection of action, inhibition and augmentation spectra in solar urticaria. Dermatology 1995;191:286–91
22. Ng JCH, Foley PA, Crouch RB, Baker CS. Changes of photosensitivity and action spectrum with time in solar urticaria. Photodermatol Photoimmunol Photomed. 2002;18:191–5
23. Hasei K, Ichihashi M. Solar urticaria: detection of action and inhibition spectra. Arch Dermatol. 1982;118:346–50
24. Horio T, Yoshioka A, Okamoto H. Production and inhibition of solar urticaria by visible light exposure. J Am Acad Dermatol. 1984;11:1094–9
25. Ichihashi M, Hasei K, Hayashibe K. Solar urticaria: further studies on the role of inhibition spectra. Arch Dermatol. 1985;121:503–7
26. Leenutaphong V. Solar urticaria induced by UVA and inhibited by visible light. J Am Acad Dermatol. 1993;29:337–40
27. Danno K, Mori N. Solar urticaria: report of two cases with augmentation spectrum. Photodermatol Photoimmunol Photomed. 2000;16:30–3
28. Horio T, Fujigaki K. Augmentation spectrum in solar urticaria. J Am Acad Dermatol. 1988;18:1189–93
29. Harber LC, Holloway RM, Wheatley VR, Baer RL. Immunologic and biophysical studies in solar urticaria. J Invest Dermatol. 1963;41:439–43
30. Rajka E. Passive transfer in light urticaria. J Allergy Clin Immunol. 1942;13:327–45
31. Torinuki W, Tagami H. Solar urticaria without inhibitory spectrum: demonstration of both circulating photoallergen and reaginic antibodies. Dermatologica 1986;173:116–9
32. Epstein S. Urticaria photogenica. Ann Allergy. 1949;7:443–57
33. Horio T, Minami K. Solar uricaria: photoallergen in a patient's serum. Arch Dermatol. 1977;113:157–60
34. Fukunaga A, Horikawa T, Yamamoto Y, Yamada Y, Nishigori C. The inhibition spectrum of solar urticaria suppresses the wheal-flare response following intradermal injection with photo-activated autologous serum but not with compound 48/80. Photodermatol Photoimmunol Photomed. 2006;22:129–32
35. Leenutaphong V, Holzle E, Plewig G. Pathogenesis and classification of solar urticaria: a new concept. J Am Acad Dermatol. 1989;21:237–40
36. Magnus IA, Jarrett A, Prankerd TAJ, Rimington C. Erythropoitic protoporphyria syndrome with solar urticaria due to protoporphyrinemia. Lancet 1961;2:448–51
37. Ichihashi M, Hasei K, Horikawa T. A case of porphyria cutanea tarda with experimental light urticaria. Brit J Dermatol. 1985;113:745–50
38. Horio T. Chlorpromazine photoallergy: coexistence of immediate and delayed type. Arch Dermatol. 1975;111:1469–71

39. Yap LM, Foley PA, Crouch RB, Baker CS. Drug-induced solar urticaria due to tetracycline. Australas J Dermatol. 2000;41:181–4
40. Kurumaji Y, Shono M. Drug-induced solar urticaria due to repinast. Dermatology 1994;188: 117–21
41. Morison WL. Solar urticaria due to progesterone compounds in oral contraceptives. Photodermatol Photoimmunol Photomed. 2003;19:155–6
42. Crow KD, Alexander E, Buck WHL, Johnson BE, Magnus IA, Porter AD. Photosensitivity due to pitch. Br J Dermatol. 1961;73:220–32
43. Tokura Y, Takigawa M, Yamauchi T, Yamada M. Solar urticaria: a case with good therapeutic response to cimetidine. Dermatologica 1986;173:224–8
44. Addo HA, Sharma SC. UVB phototherapy and photochemotherapy (PUVA) in the treatment of polymorphic light eruption and solar urticaria. Br J Dermatol. 1987;116:539–49
45. Beissert S, Stander H, Schwarz T. UVA rush hardening for the treatment of solar urticaria. J Am Acad Dermatol. 2000;42:1030–2
46. Collins P, Ferguson J. Narrow-band UVB (TL-01) phototherapy: an effective preventive treatment for the photodermatoses. Brit J Dermatol. 1995;132:956–63
47. Dawe RS, Ferguson J. Prolonged benefit following ultraviolet A for solar urticaria. Br J Dermatol. 1997;137:144–8
48. Keahey TM, Lavker RM, Kaidbey KH, Atkins PC, Zweiman BZ. Studies on the mechanism of clinical tolerance in solar urticaria. Brit J Dermatol. 1984;110:327–38
49. Ramsay CA. Solar urticaria treatment by inducing tolerance to artificial radiation and natural light. Arch Dermatol. 1977;113:1222–5
50. Parrish JA, Jaenicke KF, Morison WL, Komtaz K, Shea C. Solar urticaria: treatment with PUVA and mediator inhibitors. Brit J Dermatol. 1982;106:575–80
51. Neittaanmaki H, Jaaskelainen T, Harvima RJ, Fraki JE. Solar urticaria: demonstration of histamine release and effective treatment with doxepin. Photodermatology 1989;6:52–5
52. Edstrom DW, Ros AM. Cyclosporin A therapy for severe solar urticaria. Photodermatol Photoimmunol Photomed. 1997;13:61–3
53. Puech-Plottova I, Michel JL, Rouchouse B, Perrot JL, Dzviga C, Cambazard F. Solar urticaria: one case treated by intravenous immunoglobulin. Ann Dermatol Venereol. 2000;127:831–5
54. Mang R, Stege H, Budde MA, Ruzicja T, Krutmann J. Successful treatment of solar urticaria by extracorporeal photochemotherapy (photopheresis) – a case report. Photodermatol Photoimmunol Photomed. 2002;18:196–8
55. Collins P, Ahamat R, Green C, Ferguson J. Plasma exchange therapy for solar urticaria. Br J Dermatol. 1996;134:1093–7
56. Koranda FC. Antimalarials. J Am Acad Dermatol. 1981;4:650–5
57. Willis I, Epstein JH. Solar- vs heat-induced urticaria. Arch Dermatol. 1974;110:389–92

Cholinergic Urticaria and Exercise-Induced Anaphylaxis

5.6

Ruth A. Sabroe

Core Messages

- Cholinergic urticaria is a common type of physical urticaria, and consists of small, short-lived urticarial weals occurring after a rise in core temperature.
- Exercise-induced anaphylaxis (EIA) is a rare condition in which physical exertion, but not other causes of an increase in core temperature, causes symptoms of anaphylaxis. Sometimes food must be ingested for an attack to occur, and sometimes a specific foodstuff.
- The pathogenesis of the conditions is unclear.
- H1 antihistamines may help.
- The diseases may be both disabling and persistent.

5.6.1 Introduction: The Disease Spectrum

Cholinergic urticaria consists of small, short-lived urticarial weals occurring after a rise in core temperature. It is usually classified as one of the more common physical urticarias [1, 2], but some authors separate it from the physical urticarias, since it can also be triggered by sweating induced by emotion or eating.

Cholinergic urticaria is the most frequently occurring condition in an overlapping spectrum of transient cutaneous disorders precipitated by a rise in core temperature (Table 5.6.1) [3]. This spectrum includes: cholinergic pruritus, in which short-lived itching occurs [2, 4]; cholinergic urticaria, in which a transient itchy rash is seen [2, 5], which may sometimes, if the disease is severe enough, be associated with angio-oedema [6, 7] or the systemic symptoms of anaphylaxis [6]. There may be some overlap between cholinergic anaphylaxis [6] and exercise-induced anaphylaxis (EIA) [8, 9], but in pure EIA, anaphylactic symptoms are

R. A. Sabroe
Barnsley Hospital NHS Foundation Trust, Gawber Road, Barnsley S75 2EP, UK
e-mail: rsabroe@doctors.org.uk

T. Zuberbier et al. (eds.), *Urticaria and Angioedema*,
DOI: 10.1007/978-3-540-79048-8_5.6, © Springer Verlag Berlin Heidelberg 2010

Table 5.6.1 The disease spectrum

Cholinergic pruritus
Cholinergic urticaria ± angio-oedema ± symptoms of anaphylaxis
Exercise-induced anaphylaxis (EIA)
Persisting cholinergic erythema
Cold-induced cholinergic urticaria
Cholinergic dermographism
Localised heat urticaria

only precipitated by exercise and not by other more passive causes of an increase in core temperature or by sweating [8, 9]. In many cases of EIA, food ingestion before exercise is required for an attack to be triggered [8, 9]. Persisting cholinergic erythema has also been described, in which the patient has multiple small monomorphic red itchy macules in a widespread distribution, maximal on the upper limbs and trunk [10]. Although individual lesions last for only up to an hour, new ones constantly appear at adjacent sites so that lesions are almost always present and the rash may easily be confused with a fixed eruption, for example, urticaria pigmentosa [10]. Other rare forms of cholinergic urticaria include cold-induced cholinergic urticaria [11] and cholinergic dermographism [12], in which the characteristic weals of cholinergic urticaria occur after a reduction in core temperature or stroking of the skin, respectively [11, 12].

This chapter will concentrate mainly on cholinergic urticaria (Sect. 5.6.2) and then outline the features of EIA (Sect. 5.6.3).

5.6.2 Cholinergic Urticaria

5.6.2.1 Epidemiology

Cholinergic urticaria occurs most frequently in young adults, and equally in both sexes [2, 13]. In a study of 493 high school and university students [13], 11.2% had symptoms of cholinergic urticaria, albeit some very mild, with the highest prevalence of 20% in the 26–28-year age group. In a smaller study of 35 patients with cholinergic urticaria [5], most developed symptoms between the age of 10 and 30 years, and in another study the average age of onset was 16 years [2]. Familial cases are rare but have been reported [14].

5.6.2.2 Pathogenesis

The pathogenesis of cholinergic urticaria is poorly understood. It is thought that mast cell degranulation and histamine release are implicated, since an elevation of histamine levels in venous blood has been reported in some patients as the rash develops [15–17].

Acetylcholine released from local sympathetic nerve endings supplying sweat glands or their vascular plexuses also appears to be involved, since the cholinergic receptor antagonist scopolamine, when applied topically or taken orally, can suppress weal formation in patients with cholinergic urticaria [10, 12, 18, 19]. However, the relationship between acetylcholine and weal formation is speculative. Acetylcholine has been shown to be able to induce degranulation of rat mast cells [20], but its effects on human skin mast cells are not known. However, there was no difference in the response to intradermal acetylcholine between patients with cholinergic urticaria, spontaneous urticaria or atopy [21]. Additionally, no generalised disturbance of autonomic function could be demonstrated in patients with cholinergic urtciaria [21].

Finally, one study suggested that a type I hypersensitivity reaction to sweat might be the cause [22]. However, cholinergic urticaria can occur without sweating, since it has been reported in patients with hypohidrosis or anhidrosis, although occlusion of superficial sweat ducts has been suggested as precipitating cholinergic urticaria in such patients [23, 24].

5.6.2.3 Clinical Features

Cholinergic urticaria is induced by an increase in core body temperature, due to emotion, exercise usually to the point of sweating, eating hot or spicy food, exposure to a high ambient temperature or having a hot bath or shower [2, 3, 5]. It has also been reported in patients undergoing haemodialysis [25, 26]. In keeping with other physical urticarias, it occurs within 15–20 min of exposure to the stimulus, and lasts for up to 1 h [1, 2, 5]. Some patients have a refractory period after an attack when there is no response to further stimulus, but otherwise the urticaria recurs reproducibly each time the stimulus is applied [2]. Cholinergic urticaria not infrequently occurs with other forms of urticaria, for example, cold urticaria [1, 27] or dermographism [2].

Weals (Figs. 5.6.1 and 5.6.2) are characteristically small, and of 2–3 mm in diameter, but have a large surrounding red flare [2, 5]. Weals may be multiple and coalesce to form

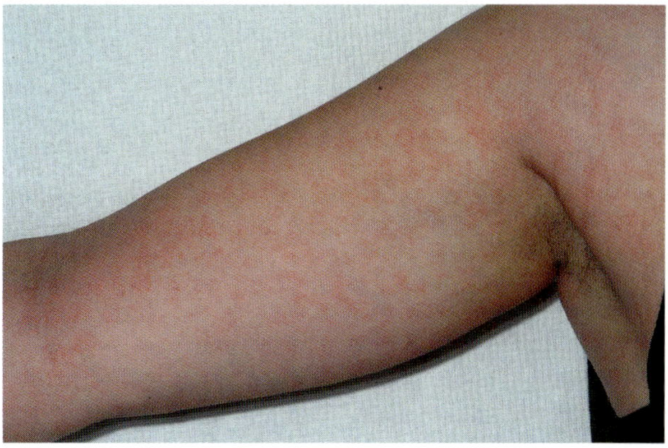

Fig. 5.6.1 Cholinergic urticaria on a patient's arm, showing multiple small typical weals in a typical distribution (ECARF, used with permission)

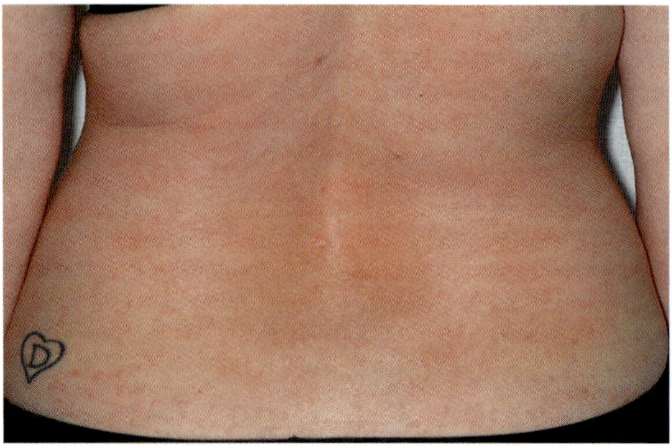

Fig. 5.6.2 Cholinergic urticaria on the same patient's back, showing multiple small typical weals, this time with more obvious surrounding large red flares (ECARF, used with permission)

plaques [2, 5]. They are most often found on the upper trunk and proximal limbs, but may be widespread [2, 5]. Weals are usually extremely itchy [2, 5].

The majority of patients present with a rash only, but if the disease is severe, systemic symptoms may occur, such as dizziness, flushing, headache, abdominal pain, nausea, diarrhoea, wheezing and breathlessness, and hypotension and fainting [2, 6, 7, 13, 17, 28]. Angio-oedema may also rarely occur [6, 7]. There is also one case report of a patient with both cholinergic urticaria and ulcerative colitis who had a transient rise in liver enzymes with each attack [29].

5.6.2.4 Confirmation of the Diagnosis

If the diagnosis is clear from the history, testing is not required. However, cholinergic urticaria can be precipitated either by exercising the patient to the point of sweating, or using a hot bath test, in which the patient is almost immersed in a bath at 42°C for 10 min [3, 30]. If the patient is prone to refractory periods or if the test is unexpectedly negative, it may be necessary to repeat the test a few days later. Treatment should be withdrawn before testing. A trained member of staff should be present throughout the test; the pulse, blood pressure and peak flow rates monitored and treatment for anaphylaxis should be available.

5.6.2.5 Differential Diagnosis

Cholinergic urticaria should be distinguished from other diseases in the same spectrum (Table 5.6.1). This can usually be done by taking a careful history, and, if there is doubt, by performing the tests listed in Sect. 5.6.2.4.

Tests for EIA are detailed in Sect. 5.6.3.

Persisting cholinergic erythema can be confirmed by carefully outlining all of the lesions in a given area with a marker pen and then reviewing the patient 1–2 h later to see if there has been any alteration in the position of the lesions. Exercise or hot bath tests will precipitate a more florid rash [10].

Cold-induced cholinergic urticaria and cholinergic dermographism can be confirmed by either a reduction in core temperature (in a specialist centre with appropriate monitoring) or by stroking the skin, respectively [11, 12].

Localised heat urticaria can be confirmed by placing a warm object against the skin, when weals will occur at the site of contact, without the need for a rise in core temperature [3].

Aquagenic urticaria and pruritus are triggered by exposure to water of any temperature. Thus, immersion of the patient in a tepid bath at 37°C will trigger aquagenic but not cholinergic symptoms and signs [3].

Dermographism may occur after bathing because of rubbing of the skin and its presence can be confirmed by gentle scratching of the skin (with pressure of less than 36 g/mm^2) [3].

Miliaria can be distinguished by the appearance of small blisters rather than weals after exercise or a hot bath test [31].

A number of other skin conditions, such as eczema, may become more itchy after bathing and can be distinguished by examining the skin before and after a hot bath test.

5.6.2.6 Treatment

Treatment is aimed at symptom control, and those patients with mild disease may not require treatment at all [13]. However, the avoidance of trigger factors may help, a cool ambient temperature may reduce attacks and the immediate application of cold water or ice may abort an attack [2]. Those patients with a refractory period may make use of this by deliberately triggering an attack 30–60 min before an important event [2]. Menthol (1–2%) in aqueous cream may provide transient relief from itching [32].

Orally, as for all other forms of urticaria, H1 antagonists are the mainstay of treatment, and many patients gain benefit from their use [2, 5, 13]. They can be taken regularly, or 1–2 h before exercise or other predictable triggers. Symptoms occur mostly during waking hours and so low-sedating antihistamines, such as cetirizine or acrivastine, are usually the most suitable [33, 34]. However, hydroxyzine has been shown to be effective and can be used if symptoms are severe or unresponsive to other antihistamines [2, 33].

In patients unresponsive to H1 antagonists, treatment becomes more difficult, and advice from a specialist centre may be sensible. There is little or no evidence to support the use of H2 antagonists, leukotriene receptor antagonists or doxepin, although a trial of their use could perhaps be justified on the basis of their beneficial effects in other forms of urticaria. Ketotifen was reported to be effective in 4 patients [16], but its use is limited by its sedative and other side effects. There are also case reports or small studies demonstrating the successful use of beta blockers [35, 36], scopolamine [18, 19], danazol [4, 37, 38], UVB [39] and prednisolone [13].

5.6.2.7 Prognosis

Cholinergic urticaria, like other forms of urticaria, can lead to high levels of disability and a marked impairment of quality of life [40]. Most patients adapt their lifestyle, but symptoms may persist for many years often becoming less severe over time [5]. In one study, 14% went into spontaneous remission, but 31% of patients had persistent symptoms for more than 10 years [5]. In another study, it took, on average, 7.5 years for patients to be no longer troubled by the condition, but some patients had continuing disease for up to 30 years [2].

5.6.3 Exercise-Induced Anaphylaxis

EIA is a rare condition in which physical exertion can lead to anaphylaxis. EIA is not induced by other more passive causes of an increase in core temperature nor by sweating, which distinguishes it from severe cholinergic disease [6, 8, 9].

EIA may occur after exercise alone, or the patient may need to eat either any food or a specific foodstuff prior to exercise for symptoms to occur [8, 9]. If a specific foodstuff is implicated, this is most commonly wheat, but EIA has occurred after eating foods as diverse as shellfish, onions, grapes, oranges, apples or peaches [8, 41–45]. Rarely eating specific foodstuffs (celery [46] or tomatoes [47]) immediately after, rather than before, exercise may cause symptoms [46, 47]. Aspirin intake before exercise may enhance attacks [8, 9, 41]. The condition appears to be more common in atopics [8, 9, 41], and one familial case has been reported [48]. A single case of cold-dependent EIA has also been reported [49].

The sex ratio is not clear. In a report of 16 patients [9], 11 were males, whereas in another report of 11 patients [8], only 4 were males. Similarly, the age of onset is unclear, although the average age at which the patients were assessed in these two studies was 24 years (range 12–54 years) [9] and 26.3 years (range 18–43 years) [8], respectively, with many patients having had the condition for several years.

It has been shown that mast cell degranulation occurs during attacks [50], and a rise in plasma histamine has also been reported [8, 42].

Symptoms include pruritus, urticaria (sometimes of cholinergic type, sometimes not), flushing, angio-oedema, cough, dyspnoea, wheeze, choking with respiratory distress, nasal discharge, diarrhoea, nausea, colic, headache, vertigo, tinnitus, hypotension and collapse [8, 9]. Symptoms may last from 30 min to 4 h, with headache persisting for 24–74 h [9].

The history may be sufficient to make the diagnosis, but if there is confusion with other causes of collapse associated with exercise, the patient can be exercised with ECG monitoring on a Bruce protocol with a cardiologist present and with treatment for anaphylaxis available [42]. It may be necessary to repeat the test before and after eating. Prick tests or measurement of specific IgE antibodies to individual foodstuffs when implicated may be positive, but not always [8, 41, 42, 46].

Treatment is aimed at the avoidance of exercise of sufficient intensity to provoke an attack [9] and, if relevant, the avoidance of eating food generally or specific foodstuffs before exercising. Aspirin and non-steroidal anti-inflammatory drugs should also be avoided before exercise [8, 9, 41]. H1 antihistamines may raise the threshold for an attack and so may be tried as prophylaxis [9]. For an actual attack, the usual emergency treatment for anaphylaxis should be provided, including intramuscular adrenaline, antihistamines, perhaps steroids and oxygen, with airway and circulatory support available if required [9, 51]. It may be helpful for patients to carry adrenaline for self-injection and to wear Medic Alert bracelets.

The problem tends to persist, and in a publication in 1999, patients had symptoms for an average of 10 years [52]. Subjects reported a reduction in the frequency of attacks over time and 41% had been attack-free for the last year, although this may largely have been attributable to altered bchaviour [52].

5.6.4 Take Home Pearls

- Cholinergic urticaria and related conditions, including EIA, form a spectrum of transient disorders precipitated by a rise in core temperature, exercise or sweating.
- The symptoms of cholinergic urticaria may be mild, but if severe the patient may suffer from a marked impairment of quality of life.
- H1 antihistamines form the mainstay of treatment, but if the disease is unresponsive it can be very difficult to find a successful alternative.
- These disorders may persist for many years.

References

1. Jorizzo JL, Smith EB. The physical urticarias: an update and review. Arch Dermatol. 1982; 118:194–201
2. Moore-Robinson M, Warin RP. Some clinical aspects of cholinergic urticaria. Br J Dermatol. 1968;80:794–9
3. Black AK, Lawlor F, Greaves MW. Consensus meeting on the definition of physical urticarias and urticarial vasculitis. Clin Exp Dermatol. 1996;21:424–6
4. Berth-Jones J, Graham-Brown RA. Cholinergic pruritus, erythema and urticaria: a disease spectrum responding to danazol. Br J Dermatol. 1989;121:235–7
5. Hirschmann JV, Lawlor F, English JSC, et al Cholinergic urticaria. A clinical and histologic study. Arch Dermatol. 1987;123:462–7
6. Kaplan AP, Natbony SF, Tawil AP, et al Exercise-induced anaphylaxis as a manifestation of cholinergic urticaria. J Allergy Clin Immunol. 1981;68:319–24
7. Lawrence CM, Jorizzo JL, Kobza-Black A, et al Cholinergic urticaria with associated angiooedema. Br J Dermatol. 1981;105:543–50
8. Dohi M, Suko M, Sugiyama H, et al Food-dependent, exercise-induced anaphylaxis: a study on 11 Japanese cases. J Allergy Clin Immunol. 1991;87:34–40
9. Sheffer AL, Austen KF. Exercise-induced anaphylaxis. J Allergy Clin Immunol. 1980;66:106–11
10. Murphy GM, Black AK, Greaves MW. Persisting cholinergic erythema: a variant of cholinergic urticaria. Br J Dermatol. 1983;109:343–8
11. Kaplan AP, Garofalo J. Identification of a new physically induced urticaria: cold-induced cholinergic urticaria. J Allergy Clin Immunol. 1981;68:438–41
12. Mayou SC, Kobza Black A, Eady RA, et al Cholinergic dermographism. Br J Dermatol 1986; 115:371–7
13. Zuberbier T, Althaus C, Chantraine-Hess S, et al Prevalence of cholinergic urticaria in young adults. J Am Acad Dermatol. 1994;31:978–81

14. Onn A, Levo Y, Kivity S. Familial cholinergic urticaria. J Allergy Clin Immunol. 1996; 98: 847–9
15. Kaplan AP, Beaven MA. In vivo studies of the pathogenesis of cold urticaria, cholinergic urticaria, and vibration-induced swelling. J Invest Dermatol. 1976;67:327–32
16. McClean SP, Arreaza EE, Lett-Brown MA, et al Refractory cholinergic urticaria successfully treated with ketotifen. J Allergy Clin Immunol. 1989;83:738–41
17. Soter NA, Wasserman SI, Austen KF, et al Release of mast-cell mediators and alterations in lung function in patients with cholinergic urticaria. N Engl J Med. 1980;302:604–8
18. Tsunemi Y, Ihn H, Saeki H, et al Cholinergic urticaria successfully treated with scopolamine butylbromide. Int J Dermatol. 2003;42:850
19. Ujiie H, Shimizu T, Natsuga K, et al Severe cholinergic urticaria successfully treated with scopolamine butylbromide in addition to antihistamines. Clin Exp Dermatol. 2006;31:588–9
20. Fantozzi R, Masini E, Blandina P, et al Release of histamine from rat mast cells by acetylcholine. Nature 1978;273:473–4
21. Murphy GM, Smith SE, Smith SA, et al Autonomic function in cholinergic urticaria and atopic eczema. Br J Dermatol. 1984;110:581–6
22. Adachi J, Aoki T, Yamatodani A. Demonstration of sweat allergy in cholinergic urticaria. J Dermatol Sci. 1994;7:142–9
23. Itakura E, Urabe K, Yasumoto S, et al Cholinergic urticaria associated with acquired generalized hypohidrosis: report of a case and review of the literature. Br J Dermatol. 2000;143: 1064–6
24. Kobayashi H, Aiba S, Yamagishi T, et al Cholinergic urticaria, a new pathogenic concept: hypohidrosis due to interference with the delivery of sweat to the skin surface. Dermatology 2002;204:173–8
25. Confino-Cohen R, Goldberg A, Magen E, et al Hemodialysis-induced rash: a unique case of cholinergic urticaria. J Allergy Clin Immunol. 1995;96:1002–4
26. Morel V, Hauser C. Generalized cholinergic heat urticaria induced by hemodialysis. Kidney Int. 2006;70:230
27. Sigler RW, Levinson AI, Evans R III, et al Evaluation of a patient with cold and cholinergic urticaria. J Allergy Clin Immunol. 1979;63:35–8
28. Kounis NG, MacMahon RG. Cholinergic urticaria with systemic manifestations. Ann Allergy. 1975;35:243–5
29. Niv Y, Elkan I, Fraser GM. Transient hepatocellular injury during attacks of cholinergic urticaria. Isr J Med Sci. 1997;33:50–2
30. Commens CA, Greaves MW. Tests to establish the diagnosis in cholinergic urticaria. Br J Dermatol. 1978;98:47–51
31. La Shell MS, Tankersley MS, Guerra A. Pruritus, papules, and perspiration. Ann Allergy Asthma Immunol. 2007;98:299–302
32. Bromm B, Scharein E, Darsow U, et al Effects of menthol and cold on histamine-induced itch and skin reactions in man. Neurosci Lett. 1995;187:157–60
33. Kobza Black A, Aboobaker J, Gibson JR, et al Acrivastine versus hydroxyzine in the treatment of cholinergic urticaria. A placebo-controlled study. Acta Derm Venereol. 1988;68:541–4
34. Zuberbier T, Munzberger C, Haustein U, et al Double-blind crossover study of high-dose cetirizine in cholinergic urticaria. Dermatology 1996;193:324–7
35. Ammann P, Surber E, Bertel O. Beta blocker therapy in cholinergic urticaria. Am J Med. 1999;107:191
36. Conway MJ. A beta-adrenergic blocker for cholinergic urticaria. Practitioner 1982; 226: 940–1
37. La Shell MS, England RW. Severe refractory cholinergic urticaria treated with danazol. J Drugs Dermatol. 2006;5:664–7

38. Wong E, Eftekhari N, Greaves MW, et al Beneficial effects of danazol on symptoms and laboratory changes in cholinergic urticaria. Br J Dermatol. 1987;116:553–6
39. Hannuksela M, Kokkonen EL. Ultraviolet light therapy in chronic urticaria. Acta Derm Venereol. 1985;65:449–50
40. Poon E, Seed PT, Greaves MW, et al The extent and nature of disability in different urticarial conditions. Br J Dermatol. 1999;140:667–71
41. Aihara M, Miyazawa M, Osuna H, et al Food-dependent exercise-induced anaphylaxis: influence of concurrent aspirin administration on skin testing and provocation. Br J Dermatol. 2002;146:466–72
42. Buchbinder EM, Bloch KJ, Moss J, et al Food-dependent, exercise-induced anaphylaxis. JAMA. 1983;250:2973–4
43. Morimoto K, Tanaka T, Sugita Y, et al Food-dependent exercise-induced anaphylaxis due to ingestion of orange. Acta Derm Venereol. 2004;84:152–3
44. Morimoto K, Hara T, Hide M. Food-dependent exercise-induced anaphylaxis due to ingestion of apple. J Dermatol. 2005;32:62–3
45. Perez-Calderon R, Gonzalo-Garijo MA, Fernandez de Soria R. Exercise-induced anaphylaxis to onion. Allergy 2002;57:752–3
46. Kidd JM III, Cohen SH, Sosman AJ, et al Food-dependent exercise-induced anaphylaxis. J Allergy Clin Immunol. 1983;71:407–11
47. Caffarelli C, Zinelli C, Trimarco G, et al Angio-oedema in a child due to eating tomatoes after excercise. Br J Dermatol. 2005;31:294–5
48. Grant JA, Farnam J, Lord RA, et al Familial exercise-induced anaphylaxis. Ann Allergy. 1985;54:35–8
49. Ii M, Sayama K, Tohyama M, et al A case of cold-dependent exercise-induced anaphylaxis. Br J Dermatol. 2002;147:368–70
50. Sheffer AL, Tong AK, Murphy GF, et al Exercise-induced anaphylaxis: a serious form of physical allergy associated with mast cell degranulation. J Allergy Clin Immunol. 1985;75: 479–84
51. Chamberlain D. Emergency medical treatment of anaphylactic reactions. Project Team of the Resuscitation Council (UK). J Accid Emerg Med. 1999;16:243–7
52. Shadick NA, Liang MH, Partridge AJ, et al The natural history of exercise-induced anaphylaxis: survey results from a 10-year follow-up study. J Allergy Clin Immunol. 1999;104: 123–7

Contact Urticaria

5.7

Jürgen Grabbe

Core Messages

- Contact urticaria is defined as wheals following contact of substances with the skin.
- The etiology of contact urticaria can be nonimmunologic or immunologic.
- Common inducers of nonimmunologic contact urticaria are plants, animals, and direct histamine liberators e.g., spices, fragrances, or drugs.
- The majority of immunologic contact urticaria cases are IgE-mediated.
- Common inducers of allergic contact urticaria are animal products, plants, foods, and drugs.

5.7.1 Etiology and Pathogenesis

There are many clinical settings in which urticaria develops as a result of contact with an exogenous agent. In such instances, the urticaria is initially at least localized to the areas of contact and thus often asymmetric. In general, one can distinguish between two types of contact urticaria: Nonimmunologic Contact Urticaria and Immunologic or Allergic Contact Urticaria. The nonimmunologic contact urticaria can occur on first exposure to a given substance in the many individuals who come in contact with the material. It is generally limited to the skin and only rarely delayed. The typical causes range from plants over animals to chemicals [1].

Many *plants* contain toxins in their leaves or other parts that are introduced into the skin via fine hairs and elicit wheals. The classic example is the stinging nettle (*Urtica*) (Fig. 5.7.1).

J. Grabbe
Department of Deruratology, Kantonsspital Aarau, 5001 Aarau, Switzerland
e-mail: juergen.grobbe@ksa.ch

T. Zuberbier et al. (eds.), *Urticaria and Angioedema*,
DOI: 10.1007/978-3-540-79048-8_5.7,

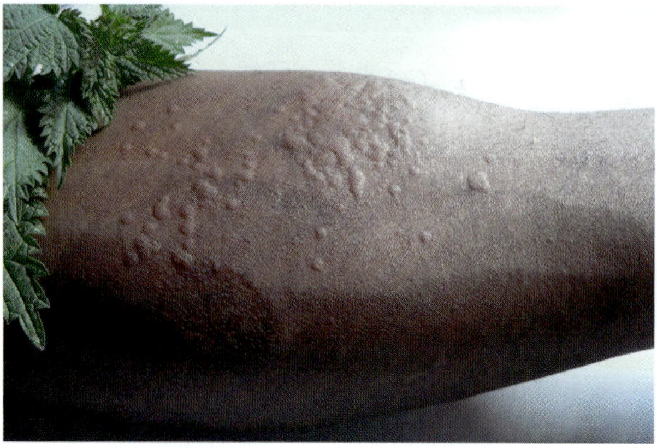

Fig. 5.7.1 Contact urticaria from *urtica dioica*

Regarding *animal elicitors*, there are a variety of jellyfish and sea anemones that cause urticaria as part of the direct action of their toxins. Also, the toxic spines of a variety of caterpillars can cause urticarial reactions. The typical scenario is hundreds of caterpillars falling from trees and affecting a number of individuals with urticarial lesions on exposed surfaces. A commonly responsible moth is the pine processionary moth [2]. While in many instances histamine is released, there is also evidence for an IgE-mediated reaction. Patients may develop papular urticaria as allergic lesions apart from the direct contact. But many other arthropods can induce urticarial reactions as well, usually around the site of their bites.

Included as causative agents are bees, wasps, hornets, spiders, bed bugs, fleas, mosquitoes, and ants. When the reaction is only toxic, it usually resolves rapidly. Often there is an allergic aspect, manifested by the evidence of IgE involvement, urticaria at distant sites, and persistence of the reaction.

Scabies can also present with urticaria, but in this case it usually represents sensitization.

Third, there are a number of substances not viewed as toxins that can directly cause release of histamine from mast cells and are therefore grouped under the name of *histamine Liberators*. When they are applied topically, they produce localized urticaria. Included in this group are some fish; however, the majority of food reactions is actually allergic. Other selected examples are spices (mustard, cinnamon), fragrances (balsam of Peru, cinnamon aldehyde), medications (menthol, camphor, capsaicin, nicotinic acid esters, benzocaine, alcohol, bacitracin, polymyxin), metals (mainly cobalt salts), preservatives (benzoic acid, sorbic acid, formaldehyde), and many others.

The allergic contact urticaria can be viewed as a rapid-acting relative of allergic contact dermatitis. Patients are sensitized to a given compound and when it is applied to the skin, there is an IgE-mediated immediate urticarial reaction. Most materials that induce urticaria are proteins, but smaller molecules can act as haptens in producing an allergic contact urticaria. Associated systemic reactions are seen, so that the synonym "contact urticaria syndrome" has been proposed. In rare cases, the contact urticaria may have a delayed onset

(4–6 h) or convert into a more typical allergic contact dermatitis. There exist various possible contact allergens.

Animal Products like hair, blood, and other products may be responsible. Amniotic fluid is a major problem in veterinarians, who traditionally deliver baby animals without wearing gloves [3]. Reactions to gelatin, fish bait from insect larvae, and silk may fit into this category. As mentioned earlier, most of the insect toxins can sensitize individuals, later causing allergic reactions.

Plant Products can also trigger allergic reactions. The most important vegetable agent today is latex. As the use of protective gloves had increased, the incidence of latex allergy in healthcare workers had risen dramatically and reached probably over 10% in most societies. Patients with spina bifida are at particular risk. Those with latex allergy are also at the risk of immediate reactions to various foods, such as bananas and tomatoes. The use of no-powder and high-quality gloves containing lower amounts of latex proteins has however greatly reduced the frequency of sensitization in the last years [4].

Almost every *food* has been described to produce immediate allergic reactions. Examples are spices, potatoes, asparagus, tomatoes, onions, garlic, peanuts, dairy products, fish meal, and honey. Protein contact dermatitis is a type of immunologic contact urticaria seen almost exclusively in food handlers, who develop itching, erythema, urticaria within 30–60 min of handling certain fresh foods and later even dyshidrosiform changes [5]. Diagnosis can be very difficult in such patients, as some react only by patch test in already damaged skin, others will have a positive prick test, and yet others will only have a positive RAST.

Food allergens and plants may also elicit symptoms of the lips, tongue, oral mucosa, and pharynx. Adults merely complain of tingling or itching after eating a variety of fruit or vegetables, including apples, nuts, and carrots [6]. Often there is a cross-reaction with birch pollen. Swelling of the lips may occur in children fed with typical allergens like cow's milk, hen egg, soy, or wheat.

Frequent sensitizers are found under *pharmaceuticals*; topical antibiotics are one example. Penicillin is so allergenic that it is not used topically. Not only patients but also nurses and other healthcare workers are at risk. Phenothiazines, pyrazolones, nitrogen mustard, benzocaine, and even some corticosteroids have been responsible for acute allergic reactions.

A long list of other miscellaneous triggers includes ammonium persulfate bleach (used by beauticians), epoxies, acrylics, some metal salts (e.g., platinum), and enzymes.

5.7.2 Clinical Findings

Immediate urticaria at a localized site of contact is the typical picture. Protein contact urticaria is typically seen in food handlers on the hands and may develop into dyshidrotic dermatitis. Another special variant is perioral erythema and swelling seen in atopic patients, especially children with food allergies.

5.7.3 Diagnostic Approach

The relationship between exposure and reaction is so temporally and spatially restricted that most patients can identify the villain. If not, a step-wise diagnostic approach is recommended:

- Open application or patch test with occlusion for only 20 min in intact and previously damaged skin; read after 30 min and after 24 h if protein contact dermatitis is suspected.
- Prick or scratch test.
- Controlled exposure, such as wearing latex gloves.
- Specific IgE antibodies can be sought with RAST or other methods.

5.7.4 Course and Prognosis

Most nonallergic reactions are a nuisance at worst, because large amounts of toxins are unlikely to be introduced. Unlucky exposure to a jellyfish is a possible exception. On the other hand, an allergic reaction is unpredictable. There are overlaps between localized allergic contact urticaria, allergic contact dermatitis, widespread urticaria, and systemic symptoms; culminating, for example, in shock in a patient with latex allergy operated on by a surgeon wearing latex gloves.

5.7.5 Therapy

The main treatment is avoidance. Antihistamines are helpful in those cases that are IgE-mediated but usually pretreatment is required. Desensitization is difficult; success has been reported in patients with contact urticaria to latex or seminal fluid. Also, patients with oral symptoms to fruit and vegetables may profit from specific immunotherapy, such as with birch pollen antigen for hay fever.

5.7.6 Take Home Pearls

- Contact urticaria is frequent.
- Diagnostic procedures include prick test, patch test with reading after 20 min and 24 h, and specific IgE antibodies.
- The main treatment is avoidance of eliciting factors.

References

1. Wakelin SH. Contact urticaria. Clin Exp Dermatol. 2001;26:132–6
2. Vega J, Vega JM, Moneo I, Armentia A, Caballero ML, Miranda A. Occupational immunologic contact urticaria from pine processionary caterpillar (Thaumetopoea pityocampa): experience in 30 cases. Contact Dermatitis. 2004;50:60–4
3. Valsecchi R, Leghissa P, Cortinovis R. Occupational contact dermatitis and contact urticaria in veterinarians. Contact Dermatitis. 2003;49:167–8
4. Allmers H, Schmengler J, John SM. Decreasing incidence of occupational contact urticaria caused by natural rubber latex allergy in German health care workers. J Allergy Clin Immunol. 2004;114:347–51
5. Amaro C, Goossens A. Immunological occupational contact urticaria and contact dermatitis from proteins: a review. Contact Dermatitis. 2008;58:67–75
6. Konstantinou GN, Grattan CE. Food contact hypersensitivity syndrome: themucosal contact urticaria paradigm. Clin Exp Dermatol. 2008;33:383–9

Urticarial Syndromes and Autoinflammation

5.8

Kanade Shinkai and Kieron S. Leslie

Core Messages

> › Recent genetic studies of urticaria have revealed distinct molecular pathways underlying different types of urticaria, and have defined several urticarial syndromes associated with autoinflammation. Although the cutaneous presentation of urticarial syndromes is strikingly similar, many of these syndromes involve diverse features of systemic inflammation and multiorgan involvement. These autoinflammatory syndromes lack the typical autoreactive lymphocytes or autoantibodies seen in autoimmune disease, instead marked by aberrant cytokine regulation. To date, the genetic basis for six autoinflammatory syndromes with urticaria has been elucidated and are reviewed here. Therapies targeting cytokine pathways have provided promising treatment for many of these autoinflammatory diseases.

Abbreviations

AA serum amyloid; *ANA* antinuclear antibody; *CAPS* cryopyrin-associated periodic syndrome; *CBC* complete blood count; *CNS* central nervous system; *CRP* C-reactive protein; *CSA* cyclosporine; *DIF* direct immunofluorescence; *ESR* erythrocyte sedimentation rate; *FCAS* familial cold-induced autoinflammatory syndrome; *FMF* familial Mediterranean fever; *HIDS* hyperimmunoglobulin D with periodic fever syndrome; *HLA* human leukocyte antigen; *HSP* Henoch Schonlein purpura; *IL* interleukin; *IgD/IgE/IgM* immunoglobulin D/E/M; *IFE* immunofixation electrophoresis; *MWS* Muckle–Wells syndrome; *NOMID* neonatal onset multi-system inflammatory disorder; *NSAIDs* nonsteroidal anti-inflammatory drugs; *SPEP* serum protein electrophoresis; *TNF* tumor necrosis factor; *TRAPS* tumor necrosis factor receptor-associated periodic syndrome

K. Shinkai (✉)
Departments of Dermatology, University of California, San Francisco, 1701 Divisadero Street, San Francisco, CA 94115, USA
e-mail: shinkaik@derm.ucsf.edu

T. Zuberbier et al. (eds.), *Urticaria and Angioedema*,
DOI: 10.1007/978-3-540-79048-8_5.8,

5.8.1 Distinct Molecular Pathways Underlying Urticarial Syndromes Associated with Autoinflammation

Within the spectrum of urticaria, there is a subset of urticarial disease observed in association with autoinflammatory syndromes, a distinct class of syndromes of systemic inflammation. These diseases are almost always marked by fever, dysregulation of cytokines, organ-specific inflammation, amyloidosis, and cutaneous manifestations [1, 2]. Unlike autoimmunity, there is no evidence of associated autoantibody production or autoreactive lymphocytes. These diseases can be inherited or acquired, and the identification of a genetic basis in several of these diseases has revealed novel molecular pathways underlying inflammatory pathways in skin, distinct from previously appreciated models such as histamine-, IgE-, or Fc receptor-mediated signaling. This paradigm shift in the pathophysiology of urticaria, in turn, has resulted in the development of novel therapeutic strategies targeting the treatment of urticaria. Classification of these diseases, however, remains a challenging task, one that continues to evolve with the rapidly expanding knowledge of the molecular pathways leading to urticaria.

5.8.2 Urticaria: Inherited or Acquired

The urticaria seen in association with autoinflammatory syndromes often bears a neutrophilic predominance, with dermal infiltration by neutrophils or neutrophils predominating at adnexal structures. The differential diagnosis of neutrophilic urticaria includes both inherited and acquired diseases, and is outlined in Table 5.8.1. Neutrophilic dermatoses represent approximately 10% of all urticaria and are an important consideration in the differential of atypical urticaria, especially that associated with systemic illness or neutrophilic infiltrate on biopsy. Urticaria has been reported as a presenting cutaneous manifestation of neutrophilic dermatoses including urticarial vasculitis [3], Sweet's disease [4], and Behcet's disease [5].

5.8.3 Familial Urticarial Syndromes

Familial urticarias associated with autoinflammatory syndromes may be suspected in the presence of a positive family history, neonatal onset, systemic involvement with or without end-organ damage, periodic fevers, amyloidosis, neutrophilic predominance, and nonpruritic quality [1]. Like all neutrophilic urticaria, these are often unresponsive or resistant to treatment, and persist or recur over many years.

Several genes are now recognized in association with autoinflammatory syndromes; these encode mediators in pathways of inflammation and cytokine production. Familial

Mediterranean Fever (FMF) and Cryopyrin-associated periodic syndrome (CAPS) both involve dysregulation of interleukin-1 cytokine signaling [6]. Other autoinflammatory syndromes involving cytokine dysregulation and urticaria are hereditary periodic fever syndromes such as Tumor necrosis factor receptor-associated periodic syndrome (TRAPS) and hyperimmunoglobulin D syndrome (HIDS).

Familial Mediterranean fever (FMF) is the quintessential periodic fever, accompanied by inflammation of joints, serous membranes, and cutaneous manifestations [7], and was one of the first to be elucidated at the molecular level [8, 9]. The classic skin finding in this autosomal recessive syndrome is erysipelas-like acral erythema [10]; however, atypical urticaria [11] and palpable purpura – both nonspecific and in the setting of Henoch–Schonlein purpura – have also been recently described [12]. The mutation in the *MEFV* gene, which encodes pyrin (marenostrin), leads to an elevated IL-1 cytokine production [13].

TRAPS (tumor necrosis factor receptor-associated periodic syndrome) is an autosomal dominant syndrome of recurrent periodic fevers, abdominal pain, urticarial skin lesions, and myalgia, associated with mutations in the TNF receptor-1 gene (TNFRSF-1A gene) [14]. In a study of 25 patients with a clinical and molecular diagnosis of TRAPS [15], skin eruptions lasted a mean 13 days (range 4–21 days); migratory erythematous macules and patches, edematous dermal plaques were the most common skin manifestations. Associated findings included conjunctivitis, periorbital edema, arthralgias, pleurisy, and headache. Skin biopsy revealed superficial and deep perivascular and interstitial infiltrate of lymphocytes and monocytes. Rare cutaneous eruptions, such as vasculitis and panniculitis, have been reported [16].

HIDS (hyperimmunoglobulinemia D syndrome) is an autosomal recessive syndrome of sporadic high fevers, abdominal symptoms, intermittent morbilliform rash, headaches, serositis, and arthralgias, seen in association with markedly elevated serum IgD levels and increased number of IgD-positive plasma cells in the bone marrow [17–19]. Lymphadenopathy, especially cervical, is a common feature. Episodes lasted on average 3–7 days, occurring every 4–8 weeks, and are linked to mutations in the *MVK* gene that encodes mevalonate kinase. 82 percent of patients demonstrate skin lesions with periodic fevers, including 24% with urticaria [18]. Amyloidosis is a rare but reported complication [20].

Cryopyrin-associated periodic syndrome, or CAPS, is a group of related clinical diseases marked by fever, urticaria, and systemic inflammation associated with mutations in the *CIAS-1* gene (cold-induced autoinflammatory syndrome 1) [21]. Prior to the discovery of the shared genetic basis, CAPS was initially described as three distinct clinical diseases: Familial cold-induced autoinflammatory syndrome (FCIAS), Muckle–Wells syndrome (MWS), and Neonatal-onset multisystem inflammatory disease (NOMID, also known as CINCA) [22]. The recognition of their shared genetic basis and pathophysiology, and their overlapping clinical features, has led to the grouping of the diseases associated with *CIAS-1* mutations into a single autoinflammatory syndrome [23]. The mildest of the three, FCIAS, is marked by fever, cold-induced urticaria, and arthralgia. MWS bears the classic triad of urticaria, deafness, and amyloidosis. NOMID presents at birth with neonatal-onset urticaria with later development of protean manifestations of central nervous system (CNS) disease and severe arthropathy [24]. The urticarial rash observed in all three diseases is indistinguishable, and displays interstitial neutrophilia and neutrophilic eccrine hidadrenitis on biopsy. The *CIAS-1* gene encodes cryopyrin, also known as Nalp3, a protein member

Table 5.8.1 Differential diagnosis of neutrophilic urticaria

Disease	Skin	Systemic features
Cryopyrin-associated periodic syndrome (CAPS) Autosomal dominant	Atypical urticarial eruption	Fevers, arthralgias
FCAS (MIM120100) mild	Cold-induced atypical urticarial eruption	Fevers, arthralgia
MWS (MIM191900) moderate	Daily atypical urticarial eruption with onset at birth	Fevers, sensorineural deafness, arthralgia, renal amyloidosis
NOMID (MIM607115) severe	Daily atypical urticarial eruption with onset at birth	Fevers. amyloidosis, arthropathy, neurologic (chronic aseptic meningitis, papilledema)
FMF (MIM249100) Autosomal recessive	Intermittent erysipelas-like erythema at acral sites, atypical urticaria, HSP and nonspecific purpuric lesions	Fevers, peritonitis, arthritis, pleuritis, renal amyloidosis, meningitis, pleurisy
TRAPS (MIM142680) Autosomal dominant	Intermittent migratory erythematous macules and papules overlying areas of myalgia, edematous plaques, purpura	Fevers, abdominal pain, pleurisy
HIDS (MIM260920) Autosomal recessive	Intermittent morbilliform rash	Arthralgia, severe abdominal pain, lymphadenopathy
Stills' disease Acquired	Evanescent erythematous eruption	Seronegative arthritis, organomegaly, CNS, ocular signs
Sweet's disease Acquired	Juicy, erythematous well demarcated plaques, bullae	Fever, arthralgias, ocular involvement
Pyoderma gangrenosum Acquired	Ulceration with violaceous, undermined border	Fever, pain, arthralgias malaise
Schnitzler's disease Acquired	Painful urticaria	Fever. IgM gammopathy. Bone pain. arthralgias
Urticarial vasculitis Acquired	Painful urticaria with male predominance, heal with purpura or hyperpigmentation	Photosensitivity, arthralgias/myalgias
Behcet's disease Acquired	Recurrent oral and genital ulcer Uveitis Erythema nodosum	Vasculitis, venous occlusive disease

Duration	Gene	Gene Product	Diagnostic tests	Treatment
Daily	*CIAS1*	Cryopyrin (Nalp3)	CRP/ESR Genetic testing	Anakinra (IL-1 receptor antagonist), rilonacept, canakinumab
Daily	*CIAS1*	Cryopyrin (Nalp3)	CRP/ESR Genetic testing	Anakinra (IL-1 receptor antagonist), rilonacept, canakinumab
Daily	*CIAS1*	Cryopyrin (Nalp3)	CRP/ESR Serum amyloid A Urinalysis Creatinine Genetic testing	Anakinra (IL-1 receptor antagonist), rilonacept, canakinumab
Daily	*CIAS1*	Cryopyrin (Nalp3)	CRP/ESR Urinalysis Creatinine Neurologic evaluation Genetic testing	Anakinra (IL-1 receptor antagonist), rilonacept, canakinumab
First episode by age 20 12–72 h. Variable period between episodes	*MEFV*	Pyrin	White blood cell count (leukocytosis) CRP/ESR Serum amyloid A Urinalysis Creatinine Genetic testing	Colchicine
2–30 day attacks, average 21 days 6 episodes per year	*TNFRSF1A*	TNF receptor 1	CRP/ESR Serum amyloid A Genetic testing	Corticosteroids Etanercept Colchicine
1–2 days Six episodes per year	*MVK*	Mevalonate kinase	CRP/ESR Serum IgD Urine mevalonate Genetic testing	NSAIDs Corticosteroids Simvastatin
Acute or chronic variants	*N/A*	N/A	Rheumatoid factor ANA CRP/ESR	Methotrexate Hydroxychloroquine TNF blockade Leflunomide
Weeks to years	*N/A*	N/A	CBC Alkaline phosphatase Skin biopsy Cancer screening	Systemic corticosteroids
Chronic	*N/A*	N/A	CBC Hepatitis panel Bacterial culture Cancer screening	Intralesional steroids Systemic steroids Wound care CSA/TNF blockade
Chronic	*N/A*	N/A	CBC SPEP/IFE	Systemic corticosteroids CSA Cyclosporine Thalidomide Anakinra
Chronic	*N/A*	N/A	CBC Hepatitis panel Complement levels Skin biopsy, DIF Autoimmune serologies Chest radiograph	Antihistamines NSAIDs Colchicine Dapsone Hydroxychloroquine
Chronic	*N/A*	N/A	Slit lamp exam HLA-B*5101 Pathergy test	Dapsone Colchicine Thalidomide Corticosteroids

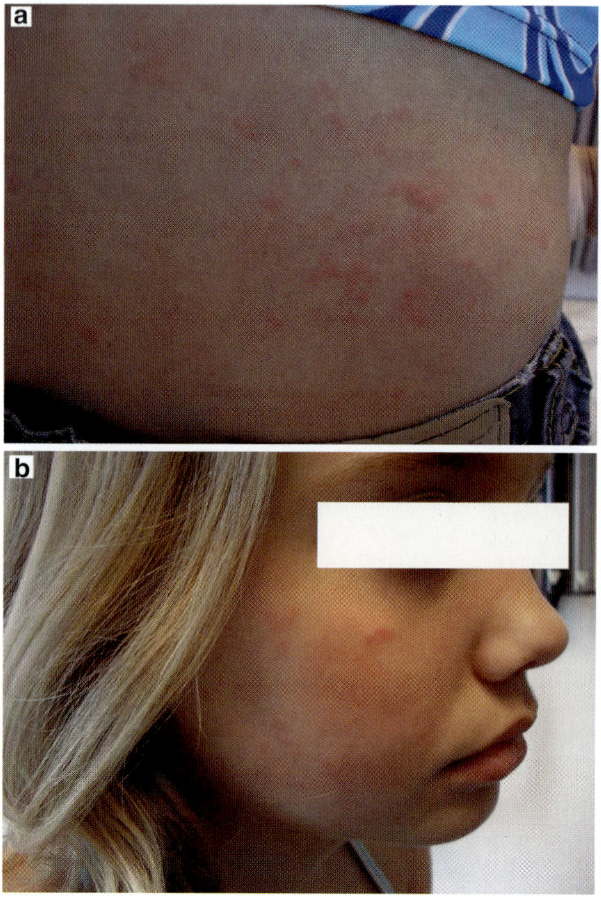

Fig. 5.8.1 Urticaria in an 8-year-old girl with cryopyrin-associated periodic syndrome (CAPS) and genetic confirmation of a mutation in the CIAS-1 gene. Her urticaria progressively worsens during the day. This patient has a history of neonatal-onset urticaria, periodic fevers, headaches with an aseptic meningitis, and sensori-neural hearing loss. She is in complete clinical remission on anakinra (IL-1 receptor antagonist) (ECARF, used with permission). (**a**) Atypical, arcuate to annular urticarial papules and plaques on the torso. (**b**) Urticarial papules on the face

of the cryopyrin inflammasome, a multi-protein regulator of IL-1 cytokine production [25]; mutations in *CIAS-1* are associated with elevations in IL-1 levels and subsequent systemic inflammation (Fig. 5.8.1).

5.8.4 Genotype–Phenotype Disparity in Autoinflammatory Disease

Despite the advances in understanding the genetic etiology of several of these autoinflammatory diseases, known mutations do not always correlate with clinical phenotype. Cryopyrin mutations are found in only 50% of patients with clinically diagnosed CAPS [26]. This disparity in genotype–phenotype is well described in CAPS, in which there are many overlapping clinical features between the three syndromes associated with CAPS. Several identical genetic mutations have been described in association with each of the

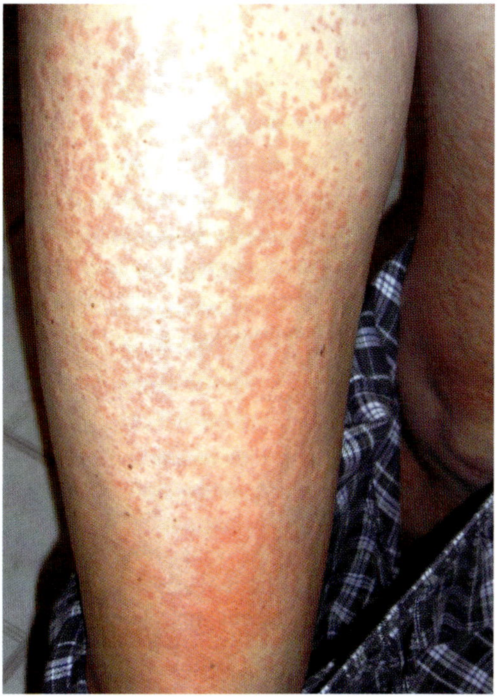

Fig. 5.8.2 Urticaria in a 33-year-old woman with lifelong urticaria, periodic fevers, headaches, and sensori-neural hearing loss. She was given a diagnosis of cryopyrin-associated periodic syndrome (CAPS) after genetic confirmation of a mutation in the CIAS-1 gene (ECARF, used with permission)

three syndromes, and cohort studies have revealed that penetrance is not 100% [27]. This disparity led to the proposal that the three associated syndromes very likely represent related diseases along a clinical spectrum, unified under a new name, CAPS [21]. The ultimate phenotypic expression of disease likely depends on environmental or genetic factors (Fig. 5.8.2).

The disparity between genotype and phenotype has also been reported in Behcet's disease and other autoinflammatory diseases. A clinical association between Behcet's and FMF was first reported in the Israeli literature [7, 28]; the association of mutations in the *MEFV* gene (the genetic mutation associated with FMF) and Behcet's disease was corroborated by several other smaller studies. In one study, 36% of patients with Behcet's disease displayed *MEFV* mutations in comparison with 11% of healthy controls [29]. A Turkish group also reported higher prevalence of *MEFV* mutations in association with Behcet's disease, especially predominant in cases with vascular involvement [12]. Mutations in the *MEFV* gene may also be a susceptibility factor to a number of other inflammatory conditions, such as Henoch–Schonlein purpura, polyarteritis nodosa, and other vasculitides; the mechanism underlying these related disorders is not understood, and penetrance is incomplete [9, 30]. However, in a Spanish cohort, neither FMF nor TRAPS are genetically associated with Behcet's disease [31]. Other autoinflammatory gene mutations have not been observed in Behcet's disease [32].

5.8.5 Nonfamilial Autoinflammatory Syndromes: Acquired or Polygenic Etiology

Atypical neutrophilic urticaria is also associated with autoinflammatory syndromes with yet unknown etiology. These are likely either acquired or polygenic in basis. Still's and Schnitzler's diseases are two examples. Still's disease is a rare autoinflammatory disorder of episodic fevers, arthralgia or arthritis, lymphadenopathy, hepatosplenomegaly, and an evanescent erythematous or morbilliform rash, sometimes with Koebner phenomenon. It is also known as systemic-onset juvenile idiopathic arthritis, or systemic juvenile rheumatoid arthritis. Urticaria has also been reported as a presenting manifestation of the disease [33]; other associated cutaneous morphologies include vesiculopustules, plaques, prurigo pigmentosa, pyoderma gangrenosum, rheumatoid nodule-like lesions on extensor surfaces, or vasculitic lesions [34–39]. Still's disease is usually divided into two clinical subsets: acute febrile systemic variant (periodic high fevers) and an oligoarthritis variant (low-grade chronic fevers). Joint disease is a major feature of Still's disease; yet, patients are typically negative for rheumatoid factor or antinuclear antibody. Systemic involvement, including organomegaly, lymphadenopathy, CNS or ocular disease, and myocarditis or pneumonitis, can be an associated morbidity. An adult-onset variant is characterized by periodic high fevers that peak later in the day, an asymptomatic morbilliform exanthem of characteristic salmon-pink papules and plaques, especially on the trunk, and arthritis with marked carpal ankylosis.

Schnitzler's disease bears chronic nonpruritic urticaria in association with recurrent fevers, arthralgias, and monoclonal IgM gammopathy. Migratory bone pain is a frequent complaint, and radiologic evidence of hyperostosis is observed in 35% of patients, especially iliac and tibial involvement. Constitutional symptoms, such as fatigue and weight loss, in association with lymphadenopathy and hepatosplenomegaly, are common features, potentially evolving into macroglobulinemia and/or hematoproliferative disease [40]. Urticaria is a chronic and prominent feature [41].

5.8.6 Diagnosis

Diagnosis can be challenging, and may require numerous testing or serial evaluations of the patient to monitor the development of associated systemic findings that suggest a disease entity. Screening tests include a complete blood count (look for marked leukocytosis), C reactive protein (CRP), erythrocyte sedimentation rate (ESR), autoimmune serologies, and immunoglobulin and complement levels. More specific tests to rule out disease entities include determinations of cytokine levels (IL-1, IL-6, TNF-alpha), serum amyloid (AA), or genetic testing for distinct gene mutations (Table 5.8.2). However, cytokine levels do not always correlate with disease activity, nor are they predictive of efficacy of anti-cytokine therapy [42]. Diagnostic maneuvers include ice cube testing, which can differentiate from cold-induced urticaria. Dermatographism is a nonspecific finding, and usually does not aid in the differentiation between typical urticarias and urticaria associated with systemic disease.

Table 5.8.2 Diagnostic evaluation of urticarias in the setting of suspected autoinflammatory disease

Screening tests
Complete blood count
C reactive protein (CRP)
Erythrocyte sedimentation rate (ESR)
Autoimmune serologies
Immunoglobulin levels
Complement levels
Creatinine
Analysis of cerebrospinal fluid
Neurologic testing (i.e., hearing test)
Urinalysis
Specific diagnostic testing
Cytokine levels (IL-1, IL-6, TNF-α)
Serum amyloid (AA)
Genetic testing for distinct gene mutations associated with autoinflammation

5.8.7 Treatment

Urticaria in the setting of autoinflammation almost always must be treated at the systemic level. Antihistamines and classical immunosuppression such as prednisone are usually not effective; there has been very strong evidence for use of cytokine immunotherapy to counterbalance the cytokine dysregulation [42–44]. As overactive IL-1 cytokine signaling is the molecular basis of CAPS, IL-1 antagonists, such as small molecule blockade (anakinra), IL-1 cytokine traps, and caspases (enzymes involved in activation of IL-1) inhibitors have been shown to be efficacious in CAPS [21, 23, 24] as well as in Schnitzler's [45], HIDS [46, 47], TRAPS [48], and FMF [49, 50]. Targeting the IL-1 cytokine pathway has been shown to not only ameliorate cutaneous manifestations but also end-organ damage such as severe renal disease secondary to amyloidosis [21, 51] and hearing loss [52, 53]. Other treatment modalities include TNF-receptor signaling blockade, which is beneficial in TRAPS [43], as well as bone marrow transplantation, which has been recently described in HIDS [54].

5.8.8 Take Home Pearls

- The genetic basis of several inherited syndromes with urticaria has recently been elucidated at a molecular and cellular level.
- Many of these urticarial syndromes are autoinflammatory in nature, involving cytokine dysregulation, and have important cutaneous manifestations in addition to systemic inflammation.

- Autoinflammatory diseases are distinct from autoimmune diseases, because they do not involve auto-antibody production or self-reactive lymphocytes.
- Therapeutics aimed at cytokine production have provided promising treatment for many autoinflammatory diseases.

References

1. Samuels J, Ozen S. Familial Mediterranean fever and the other autoinflammatory syndromes: evaluation of the patient with recurrent fever. Curr Opin Rheum. 2006;18:108–17
2. Stojanov S, Kastner DL. Familial autoinflammatory diseases: genetics, pathogenesis and treatment. Curr Opin Rheum. 2005;17:576–99
3. Sanchez-Cano D, Callejas-Rubio JL, Ortego-Centeno N, Ruiz-Villaverde R. Urticaria and angioedema in a patient with Behcet's disease treated with adalimumab. Clin Exp Rheumatol. 2006;24 5 Suppl 42:S12
4. Clemmenson OJ, Menne T, Brandrup F, Thomsen K, Lange Wantzin G. Acute febrile neutrophilic dermatosis – a marker of malignancy? Acta Derm Venereol. 1989;69(1):52–8
5. See Lee JS, Loh TH, Seow SC, Tan SH. Prolonged urticaria with purpura: the spectrum of clinical and histopathologic features in a prospective series of 22 patients exhibiting the clinical features of urticarial vasculitis. JAAD 2007;56(6):994–1005
6. Shinkai K, McCalmont TH, Leslie KS. Cryopyrin-associated periodic syndromes (CAPS) and autoinflammation. Clin Exp Dermatol. 2008;33(1):1–9
7. Kone Paut I, Dubac M, Sportouch J, Minodier P, Garnier JM, Touitou I. Phenotype-genotype correlation in 91 patients with Familial Mediterranean fever reveals a higher frequency of cutaneous features. Rheumatology 2000;39:1275–9
8. International FMF Consortium. Ancient missence mutations in a new member of the RoRet gene family are likely to cause familial Mediterranean fever. Cell. 1997;90(4):797–807
9. Tunca M, Akar S, Onen F, et al Familial Mediterranean fever (FMF) in Turkey: results of a nationwide multicenter study. Medicine 2000;84:1–11
10. Barzilai A, Langevitz P, Goldberg I, Kopolovic J, Livneh A, Pras M, Trau H. Erysipelas-like erythema of familial Mediterranean fever: clinicopathologic correlation. J Am Acad Dermatol. 2000;42 5 Pt 1:791–5
11. Alonso R, Cistero-Bahima A, Enrique E, San Miguel-Moncin MM. Recurrent urticaria as a rare manifestation of familial Mediterranean fever. J Investig Allergol Clin Immunol. 2002;12(1):60–1
12. Atagunduz P, Ergun T, Direskeneli H. MEFV mutations are increased in Behcet's disease and are associated with vascular involvement. Clin Exp Rheumatol. 2003;21: Suppl 30:S35–7
13. French FMF Consortium. A candidate gene for familial Mediterranean fever. Nat Genet. 1997; 17(1):25–31
14. McDermott MF, Aksentijevich I, Galon J, et al Germline mutations in the extracellular domains of the 55 kDa TNF receptor, TNFR1, define a family of dominantly inherited autoinflammatory syndromes. Cell 1999;97:133–44
15. Toro JR; Aksentijevich I; Hull K; Dean J; Kastner D. Tumor necrosis factor receptor-associated periodic syndrome: a novel syndrome with cutaneous manifestations. Arch Derm. 2000;136:1487–94
16. Lamprecht P, Moosig F, Adam-Klages S, Mrowietz U, Csernok E, Kirrstetter M, Ahmadi-Simab K, Schroder JO, Gross WL. Small vessel vasculitis and relapsing panniculitis in tumour necrosis factor receptor associated periodic syndrome (TRAPS). Ann Rheum Dis. 2004;63(11):1518–20
17. Drenth JPH, Boom BW, Toonstra J, van der Meer JWM. Cutaneous manifestations and histological findings in the hyperimmunoglobulinemia D syndrome. Arch Derm. 1994;130:59–65

18. Drenth JPH, Haagsma CJ, van der Meer JWM; The International Hyper-IgD Study Group. Hyperimmunoglobulinemia D and periodic fever syndrome: the clinical spectrum in a series of 50 patients. Medicine 1994;73(3):133–44
19. Drenth JPH, Cuisset L, Grateau G, Vasseur C, van de Velde-Visser SD, de Jong JGN, Beckmann JS, van der Meer JWM, Delpech M; International Hyper-IgD Study Group. Mutations in the gene encoding mevalonate kinase cause hyper-IgD and periodic fever syndrome. Nat Genet. 1999;22:178–81
20. Lachmann HJ, Goodman HJB, Andrews PA, Gallagher H, Marsh J, Breuer S, Rowczenio DM, Bybee A, Hawkins PN. AA amyloidosis complicating hyperimmunoglobulinemia D with Periodic Fever Syndrome: a report of two cases. Arthritis Rheum. 2006;54(6):2010–4
21. Leslie KS, Lachmann HJ, Bruning E, McGrath JA, Bybee A, Gallimore JR, Roberts PF, Woo P, Grattan CE, Hawkins PN. Phenotype, genotype, and sustained response to anakinra in 22 patients with autoinflammatory disease associated with CIAS-1/NALP3 mutations. Arch Dermatol 2006;142(12):1591–7
22. Shinkai K, Kilcline C, Connolly MK, Frieden IJ. The pyrin family of fever genes: unmasking genetic determinants of autoinflammatory disease. Arch Dermatol. 2006;141:242–7
23. Hawkins PN, Lachmann HJ, Aganna E, McDermott MF. Spectrum of clinical features in Muckle-Wells syndrome and response to anakinra. Arthritis Rheum. 2004;50:607–12
24. Goldbach-Mansky R, Dailey NJ, Canna SW, Gelabert A, Jones J, Rubin BI, Kim HJ, Brewer C, Zalewski C, Wiggs E, Hill S, Turner ML, Karp BI, Aksentijevich I, Pucino F, Penzak SR, Haverkamp MH, Stein L, Adams BS, Moore TL, Fuhlbrigge RC, Shaham B, Jarvis JN, O'Neil K, Vehe RK, Beitz LO, Gardner G, Hannan WP, Warren RW, Horn W, Cole JL, Paul SM, Hawkins PN, Pham TH, Snyder C, Wesley RA, Hoffmann SC, Holland SM, Butman JA, Kastner DL. Neonatal-onset multisystem inflammatory disease responsive to interleukin-1beta inhibition. NEJM 2006;355(6):581–92
25. Agostini L, Martion F, Burns K, et al NALP3 forms an IL-1 beta-processing inflammasome with increased activity in Muckle-Wells autoinflammatory disorder. Immunity 2004;20:319–25
26. Aksentijevich I, Putnam CD, Remmers EF, Mueller JL, Le J, Kolodner RD, Moak Z, Chuang M, Austin F, Goldbach-Mansky R, Hoffman HM, Kastner JL. The clinical continuum of cryopyrinopathies: novel *CIAS1* mutations in North American patients and a new cryopyrin model. Arthritis Rheum. 2007;56(4):1273–85
27. Arostegui JI, Aldea A, Modesto C, et al Clinical and genetic heterogeneity among Spanish patient with recurrent autoinflammatory syndromes associated with the CIAS1PYPAF1/Nalp3. Arthritis Rheum. 2004;50:4045–50
28. Schwartz T, Langevitz P, Zemer D, Gazit E, Pras M, Livneh A. Behcet's disease in Familial Mediterranean fever: characterization of the association between the two diseases. Semin Arthritis Rheum. 2000;29:286–95
29. Imirzalioglu N, Dursun A, Tastan B, Soysal Y, Yakicier MC. MEFV gene is a probable susceptibility gene for Behcet's disease. Scand J Rheumatol. 2005;34:56–8
30. Cattan D. MEFV mutation carriers and diseases other than Familial Mediterranean fever: proved and non-proved associations; putative biological advantage. Curr Drug Targets Inflamm Allergy. 2005;4:105–12
31. Espinosa E, Arostegui JI, Plaza S, Rius J, Cervera R, Yague J, Font J. Behcet's disease and hereditary periodic fever syndromes: casual association or causal relationship? Clin Exp Rheumatol. 2005;23 Suppl 38:S64–6
32. Kone-Paut I, Sanchez E, Le Quellec A, Manna R, Touitou I. Autoinflammatory gene mutations in Behcet's disease. Ann Rheum Dis. 2007;66:832–4
33. Salaffi F, Filosa F, Bugatti L, Maestrini MD. Urticaria as a presenting manifestation of adult-onset Still's disease. Clin Rheumatol. 2000;19(5):389–91
34. Bachmeyer C, Blum L, Petitjean B, Kemiche F, Roujeau JC, Pertuiset E. Vesiculopustules in adult-onset Still's disease. J Am Acad Dermatol. 2006;54 5 Suppl:S247–8

35. Elezoglou AV, Giamarelos-Bourboulis E, Katsilambros N, Sfikakis PP. Cutaneous vasculitis associated with mixed cryoglobulinemia in adult Still's disease. Clin Exp Rheumatol. 2003;21(3): 405–6
36. Falcini F, Tacetti G, Ermini M, Trapani S, Calzolari A, Franchi A, Cerinic MM. Methotrexate-associated appearance and rapid progression of rheumatoid nodules in systemic-onset juvenile rheumatoid arthritis. Arthritis Rheum. 1997;40(1):175–8
37. Lee JY, Yang CC, Hsu MM. Histopathology of persistent papules and plaques in adult-onset Still's disease. J Am Acad Dermatol. 2005;52(6):1003–8
38. Lubbe J, Hofer M, Chavaz P, Saurat JH, Borradori L. Adult-onset Still's disease with persistent plaques. Br J Dermatol. 1999;141(4):710–3
39. Tomaru K, Nagai Y, Ohyama N, Hasegawa M, Endo Y, Tamura A, Ishikawa O. Adult-onset Still's disease with prurigo pigmentosa-like skin eruption. J Dermatol. 2006;33(1):55–8
40. Welsh B, Tate B. Schnitzler's syndrome: report of a case with progression to Waldenstrom's macroglobulinemia. Australas J Dermatol. 1999;40(4):201–3
41. Janier M, Bonvalet D, Blanc MF, Lemarchand F, Cavelier B, Ribrioux A, Civatte J. Chronic urticaria and macroglobulinemia (Schnitzler's syndrome): report of two cases. JAAD 1989; 20(2):206–11
42. Dinarello CA. Blocking IL-1 in systemic inflammation. J Exp Med. 2005;201(9):1355–9
43. Church LD, Churchman SM, Hawkins PN, McDermott MF. Hereditary auto-inflammatory disorders and biologics. Springer Semin Immunopathol. 2006;27(4):494–508
44. Hoffman HM, Patel DD. Genomic-based therapy: targeting interleukin-1 for autoinflammatory diseases. Arthritis Rheum. 2004;50:345–9
45. De Koning HD, Bodar EJ, Simon A, van der Hilst JC, Netea MG, va der Meer JW. Beneficial response to anakinra and thalidomide in Schnitzler's syndrome. Ann Rheum Dis. 2006;65(4):542–4
46. Cailliez M, Garaix F, Rousset-Rouiere C, Bruno D, et al Anakinra is safe and effective in controlling hyperimmunoglobulinemia D syndrome-associated febrile crisis. J Inherit Metab Dis. 2006;29(6):763
47. Haas D, Hoffmann GF. Mevalonate kinase deficiencies: from mevalonic aciduria to hyperimmunoglobulinemia D syndrome. Orphanet J Rare Dis. 2006;26(1):13
48. Simon A, Bodar EJ, van der Hilst JC, van der Meer JW, Fiselier TJ, Cuppen MP, Drenth JP. Beneficial response to interleukin 1 receptor antagonist in TRAPS. Am J Med. 2004;117(3):208–10
49. Belkhir R, Moulonguet-Doleris L, Hachulla E, Prinseau J, Baglin A, Hanslik T. Treatment of familial Mediterranean fever with anakinra. Ann Intern Med. 2007;146:825–6
50. Calligaris L, Marchetti F, Tommasini A, Ventura A. The efficacy of anakinra in an adolescent with colchicines-resistant familial mediterranean fever. Eur J Pediatr. 2008;167(6):695–6
51. Thornton BD, Hoffman HM, Bhat A, Don BR. Successful treatment of renal amyloidosis due to familial cold autoinflammatory syndrome using an interleukin 1 receptor antagonist. Am J Kidney Dis. 2007;49:477–81
52. Mirault T, Launay D, Cuisset L, Hachulla E, Lambert M, Queyrel V, Quemeneur T, Morell-Dubois S, Hatron P-Y. Recovery from deafness in a patient with Muckle-Wells Syndrome treated with anakinra. Arthritis Rheumat. 2006;43(5):1697–700
53. Rynne M, Maclean C, Bybee A, McDermott MF, Emery P. Hearing improvement in a patient with variant Muckle-Wells syndrome in response to interleukin 1 receptor antagonism. Ann Rheum Dis. 2006;65:533–4
54. Neven B, Valayannopoulos V, Quartier P, Blanche S, Prieur AM, Debre M, Rolland MO, Rabier D, Cuisset L, Cavazzana-Calvo M, de Lonlay P, Fischer A. Allogeneic bone marrow transplanation in mevalonic aciduria. NEJM 2007;356:2700–3

Urticaria Vasculitis

5.9

Lluís Puig

Core Messages

- Urticaria vasculitis (UV) is a clinicopathological entity characterized by urticarial papules and plaques lasting longer than 24 h accompanied by histopathologic features of leukocytoclastic vasculitis.
- Clinical presentation of UV is characterized by urticarial papules or plaques, which can be burning or tender rather than pruritic in 33% of patients, usually persist for more than 24 h leaving residual purpura or hyperpigmentation, and are frequently associated with angioedema.
- The minimal histopathological criteria for UV have been proposed to include the presence of leukocytoclasis or fibrinoid necrosis in the lesions, irrespective of red blood cell extravasation.
- A continuum exists in the histopathologic changes of UV, which might reflect the time of evolution of lesions at the moment of biopsy.
- UV is considered to be due to deposition of immune complexes, which can be found in the circulation of 30–75% of patients.
- Patients with UV and complement activation are much more likely to have systemic disease than are patients with normocomplementemic UV. As many as 50% have moderate to severe emphysematous chronic obstructive pulmonary disease, and up to 30% have ocular inflammation, particularly uveitis.
- UV has an unpredictable course, even though the outcome is usually benign in patients with the idiopathic, normocomplementemic form of the disease.

L. Puig
Department of Dermatology, Hospital Santa Creu i Sant Pau., Universitat Autònoma de Barcelona, Sant Antoni Maria Claret 167, 08025 Barcelona, Spain
e-mail: lpuig@santpau.cat

T. Zuberbier et al. (eds.), *Urticaria and Angioedema*,
DOI: 10.1007/978-3-540-79048-8_5.9, © Springer Verlag Berlin Heidelberg 2010

5.9.1 Definition

Urticaria vasculitis (UV) is a clinicopathological entity characterized by urticarial papules and plaques of longer than 24 h duration – typically resolving with faint purpura or residual hyperpigmentation, indicating red blood cell extravasation – accompanied by histopathologic features of leukocytoclastic vasculitis in the capillaries and postcapillary venules of the skin. There should be evidence of leukocytoclasis and vessel wall destruction, which may or may not be accompanied by fibrinoid deposits.

5.9.2 Epidemiology

UV is relatively uncommon; in patients presenting with chronic urticaria, its prevalence is 5% [1–3], with women accounting for 60% [4] to 80% [5] of cases and a peak incidence in the fourth decade of life [4, 5].

5.9.3 Histopathologic Findings

The histopathology of UV often reveals most features of leukocytoclastic vasculitis, including endothelial cell injury and swelling, with disruption or occlusion of the vessel wall; extravasation of red blood cells, leukocytoclasis, fibrin deposition in and around the blood vessels; and a perivascular infiltrate composed mostly of neutrophils, even though lymphocytes can predominate in older lesions. Fibrinoid change or necrosis and particularly thrombosis are less common in UV than in fully developed lesions of palpable purpura. Some authors accept the presence a mixed inflammatory infiltrate within and around capillaries and postcapillary venules as sufficient evidence to make the diagnosis, in the absence of leukocytoclasis and fibrinoid destruction [1, 6]. Several reports suggest that a continuum exists in the histopathologic changes [7, 8], which might reflect the time of evolution of lesions at the moment of biopsy. The more severe histopathologic changes are generally associated with more severe systemic symptoms, and the minimal histopathological criteria for UV have been proposed to include the presence of leukocytoclasis or fibrinoid necrosis in the lesions, irrespective of red blood cell extravasation [1, 7].

Direct immunofluorescence studies show the presence of immunoglobulins, complement, or fibrin within vessel walls in about 70% of cases [1, 9, 10]; it is well documented that granular deposits of immunoglobulins and complement can be appreciated in the basement membrane zone in up to 79% of active lesions [4, 10]. It has been postulated that this finding might predict the eventual development of systemic lupus erythematosus (SLE) [11] or renal disease [9].

5.9.4 Pathophysiology

UV is considered to be due to deposition of immune complexes, which can be found in the circulation of 30–75% of patients [10], and may be formed by way of autoantibodies or induced exogenously by infections, such as viral hepatitis C and B, or medications (serum sickness and serum sickness-like drug reactions); in most patients, the source of antigen is never discovered [6].

The findings of sequential biopsies at 3, 10, and 24 h in a patient with exercise-induced UV have led to postulate a pathogenetic sequence: there is early (3 h) deposition of immune complexes, intense expression of E-selectin and VCAM-1, mast cell activation with release of TNF-α, and influx of eosinophils with deposition of eosinophil granule protein; an influx of neutrophils occurs at 10 h, and these cells become the predominant component of the inflammatory infiltrate at 24 h [12].

Patients with UV and complement activation are much more likely to have systemic disease than are patients with normocomplementemic UV [13]. Hypocomplementemic urticarial vasculitis syndrome (HUVS) [14], first recognized by McDuffie et al. in 1971 [15], is an uncommon autoimmune disorder in which the dominant and consistent clinical finding is recurrent to chronic UV. Angioedema occurs in up to 50% of patients and can be the first sign of HUVS [14]. As many as 50% have moderate to severe emphysematous chronic obstructive pulmonary disease (COPD), and up to 30% have ocular inflammation, particularly uveitis. Patients with HUVS are hypocomplementemic owing to persistent activation of the classical complement pathway, with decreased serum C1q and undetectable to low-normal serum levels of C3 and C4 [13, 14]. Rarely, C3 and C4 may be within normal ranges, but all such patients have decreased serum C1q, which may remain modestly decreased even when C3 and C4 return to normal during spontaneous or drug-induced remissions of HUVS [14]. IgG autoantibodies to the collagen-like region of C1q (corresponding to complement-activating C1q precipitins) are detectable using enzyme-linked immunosorbent assay in the serum of all patients with HUVS [13], but can also be found in 30–35% of unselected patients with SLE and 80% of patients with SLE and glomerulonephritis [13], and their pathogenetic contribution to either HUVS or SLE is not precisely known.

5.9.5 Clinical Features

Classically, the patients present with urticarial papules or plaques, which are burning or tender rather than pruritic in 33% of patients [4], usually persist for more than 24 h (which can be demonstrated by follow-up of outlined lesions). Angioedema (corresponding to deep vessel involvement) has been reported in up to 42% of patients [4]. Giant (>10 cm) wheals or circinate or polycyclic arrangements of lesions are less common than in urticaria. The lesions can occur anywhere on the body, especially in areas subjected to pressure. They leave residual purpura or hyperpigmentation, which can be better appreciated with the aid of diascopy or dermatoscopy. Rarely, lesions can present as livedo reticularis, erythema multiforme, or bullae [3].

5.9.6 Systemic Manifestations

Musculoskeletal symptoms are most commonly encountered and consist mainly of migratory and transient peripheral arthralgia, occurring in half the patients [4] and arthritis, which is uncommon in normocomplementemic UV but occurs in up to 50% of patients with HUVS [9]. Jaccoud's arthropathy (joint deformities similar to those in rheumatoid arthritis that can be corrected voluntarily and are not associated with joint destruction), commonly associated with rheumatic fever and SLE, has been reported in association with HUVS, and might imply an increased risk for valvular heart disease [16].

Renal involvement, usually manifested by proteinuria and microscopic hematuria, has been found to occur in 20–30% of patients with hypocomplementemia [4, 17], is quite variable histopathologically (diverse types of glomerulonephritis and interstitial nephritis) and tends to be nonprogressive [3]. Renal disease is uncommon in patients with normocomplementemic UV, but mesangial proliferative glomerulonephritis has been reported [1, 18].

Pulmonary complications include cough, dyspnea, hemoptysis, pleuritis, emphysema, COPD, and asthma; the latter two can present in approximately 17–20% [4] of hypocomplementemic patients and in 5% of normocomplementemic patients [4]. Patients with COPD and UV are frequently smokers, but UV seems to be associated with increased severity and early appearance of the pulmonary disease [19]. Leukocytoclastic vasculitis of the pulmonary vessels and release of elastase by infiltrating neutrophils can contribute to the development of emphysema in UV patients [19].

Gastrointestinal symptoms such as abdominal pain, nausea, vomiting, and diarrhea are noted by 17–30% of patients [9].

Ophthalmologic complications occur in 10% of patients with UV and 30% of patients with HUVS; they include conjunctivitis, episcleritis, iritis, or uveitis, which have been reported to occur more frequently in patients with HUVS [3].

Other infrequent systemic manifestations of UV include pericarditis, pericardial effusion, and valvular heart disease; pseudotumor cerebri and peripheral neuropathy; digital infarction and Raynaud's phenomenon, among others.

Even though constitutional symptoms can be present, fever is considered to be rare (10%) [4]. Systemic manifestations are common in patients with hypocomplementemic UV, regardless of whether it is primary or associated with an underlying disease.

Table 5.9.1 summarizes the reported causes or associations of UV. Most cases of UV have an unknown cause. Classification of idiopathic UV based on serum complement levels is useful but arbitrary, because normocomplementemic UV, hypocomplementemic UV, and HUVS might represent an evolutionary continuum; nevertheless, extended observations in more than 50 patients support the hypothesis that there is no transition among these UV subtypes [13]. Normocomplementemic UV is idiopathic in most patients, whereas

Table 5.9.1 Causes and associations of UV (adapted from ref. [3])

	Cause/association
No cause found	Idiopathic
Connective tissue diseases	SLE, Sjögren's syndrome
Immune complex diseases	Serum sickness
Drugs, medications, preservatives, and vaccines	Bacillus Calmette-Guérin, butylhydroxytoluene, butylated hydroxyanisole, cimetidine, cocaine abuse, dexfenfluramine, diltiazem, etanercept, fluoxetine, herbs, methotrexate, potassium iodide, procainamide, procarbazine
Infections	Hepatitis B virus, hepatitis C virus, Epstein–Barr virus, Lyme disease
Complement disorders	C3 deficiency, C4 deficiency, C3 nephritic factor activity
Paraproteinemia	IgM monoclonal gammopathy (Schnitzler's syndrome) IgG gammopathy
Hematologic neoplasms and diseases	Leukemia, lymphoma, polycyhemia rubra vera, idiopathic thrombocytopenic purpura, Hodgkin's disease, IgA myeloma, B-cell lymphoma
Malignancy	Malignant teratoma, metastatic adenocarcinoma of colon
Physical causes	Cold, sunlight, exercise
Other	Amyloidosis (Muckle Wells syndrome), Cogan's syndrome, striae distensae of pregnancy

secondary normocomplementemic UV has been described in patients with monoclonal gammopathy, neoplasia, and sensitivity to ultraviolet light or cold exposure [13].

5.9.7 Differential Diagnosis and Investigations

The main differential diagnosis is chronic urticaria; if UV is suspected on the basis of clinical features or associated manifestations, lesional skin should be biopsied for hematoxylin and eosin and immunofluorescent staining. Early lesions are preferred, and multiple biopsies are often required to establish the diagnosis. Evidence of leukocytoclasis and vessel wall destruction, which may be accompanied by fibrinoid deposits, as suggested by Black [1], seem to be the most acceptable criteria for the diagnosis of UV. Histologic confirmation of the diagnosis should prompt for a thorough history and physical examination. A symptom-oriented approach is useful for the evaluation of systemic involvement. Chest radiographs, pulmonary function tests, and bronchoalveolar lavage are helpful in the assessment of lung involvement. Appropriate laboratory studies should include serum antinuclear antibody, antibodies to extractable nuclear antigens, complement and cryoglobulin assays, a complete blood cell count, and measurement of renal function. Erythrocyte sedimentation rate is frequently elevated, but is nonspecific and not related to the severity of UV or to the presence of systemic involvement [10, 11]. Hypocomplementemia, as has already been discussed, is an accepted marker of systemic disease and is associated with complications. Optimal stratification of UV on the basis of serum complement levels requires measurement of serum C1q, C3, C4, and CH50 on two to three occasions during several months of observation [13]. Testing of IgG autoantibodies to the collagen-like region of C1q, if available, is helpful for investigative purposes.

5.9.8 Prognosis

UV has an unpredictable course, even though the outcome is usually benign in patients with the idiopathic, normocomplementemic form of the disease, with a disease span exceeding 12 years in the largest series reported [20]; the average duration of the disease is 3 to 4 years [4, 9]. Hypocomplementemic UV, HUVS, and SLE-associated UV have a worse prognosis [1], with COPD [20] and acute laryngeal edema [21] as common causes of morbidity and death.

5.9.9 Treatment

No therapy is universally effective, and if an underlying disease is identified, it should be the main focus of treatment. Antihistamine therapy is regularly used for symptomatic control of pruritus, but is rarely effective alone, and does not alter the course of the disease [6]. Systemic corticosteroids are the mainstay of treatment [4]. Most patients experience relapse on discontinuation of treatment and require chronic use; the dosage should be adjusted to the patient's requirement. Indomethacine, colchicine, dapsone, and antimalarials have been used to minimize corticosteroid requirement; dapsone, even as monotherapy, has been associated with long-term remissions and considered to be the drug of choice in hypocomplementemic UV [22], but is associated with potentially severe adverse effects. In many cases with severe disease involvement, corticosteroids must be combined with immunosupressants such as azathioprine, cyclophosphamide, cyclosporin, and mycophenolate mofetil [3]; methotrexate appears not to be very effective [6] and has been associated with exacerbation of UV [23]. Interferon α associated with ribavirin is an effective combination to treat hepatitis C virus infection associated with UV and cryoglobulinemia [3, 13]. Plasmapheresis, intravenous immunoglobulin, and monoclonal antibody therapies need to be evaluated further.

5.9.10 Take Home Pearls

- If UV is suspected on the basis of clinical features or associated manifestations, lesional skin should be biopsied for hematoxylin and eosin and immunofluorescent staining. Early lesions are preferred, and multiple biopsies are often required to establish the diagnosis.

- Hypocomplementemia is an accepted marker of systemic disease and is asociated with complications. Optimal stratification of UV on the basis of serum complement levels requires measurement of serum C1q, C3, C4, and CH50 on two to three occasions during several months of observation.
- Arthritis is uncommon in normocomplementemic UV but occurs in up to 50% of patients with hypocomplementemic UV syndrome.
- Pulmonary complications of UV include cough, dyspnea, hemoptysis, pleuritis, emphysema, chronic obstructive pulmonary disease, and asthma; the latter two can present in 17–20% of hypocomplementemic patients and in 5% of normocomplementemic patients.
- Normocomplementemic UV is idiopathic in most patients, but has been reported to be associated with monoclonal gammopathy, neoplasia, and sensitivity to ultraviolet light or cold exposure.
- Systemic corticosteroids are the mainstay of treatment. Dapsone, even as monotherapy, has been associated with long-term remissions and considered to be the drug of choice in hypocomplementemic UV.
- In many cases with severe disease involvement, corticosteroids must be combined with immunosupressants; methotrexate has been associated with exacerbation of UV (Figs. 5.9.1–5.9.2)

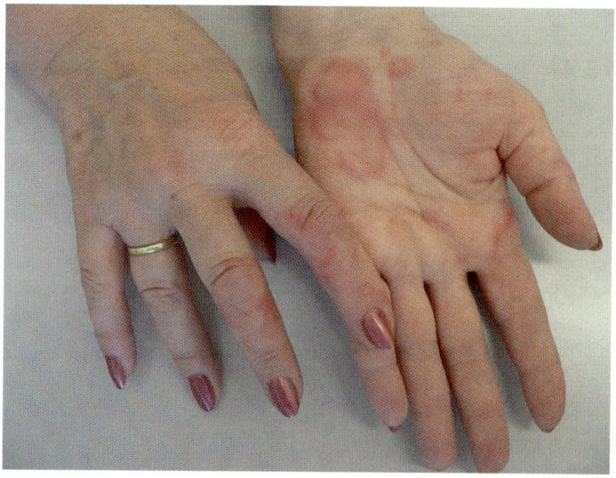

Fig. 5.9.1. Lesions in UV can be clinicaly indistinguishable from urticaria, but they usually persist for 24 hours or longer

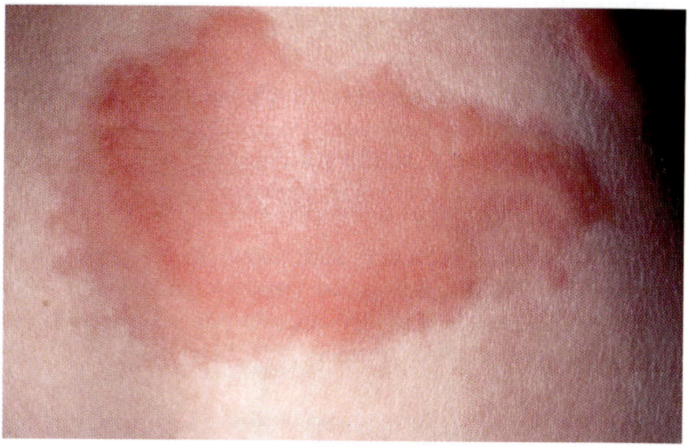

Fig. 5.9.2 The presence of purpura is suggestive of UV. Biopsy specimens from the "active" border of lesions are usually better for histopathologic confirmation of the diagnosis

References

1. Black AK. Urticarial vasculitis. Clin Dermatol. 1999;17(5):565–9
2. Champion RH. Urticaria: then and now. Br J Dermatol. 1988;119(4):427–36
3. Davis MD, Brewer JD. Urticarial vasculitis and hypocomplementemic urticarial vasculitis syndrome. Immunol Allergy Clin North Am. 2004;24(2):183–213, vi
4. Mehregan DR, Hall MJ, Gibson LE. Urticarial vasculitis: a histopathologic and clinical review of 72 cases. J Am Acad Dermatol. 1992;26(3 Pt 2):441–8
5. Aboobaker J, Greaves MW. Urticarial vasculitis. Clin Exp Dermatol. 1986;11(5):436–44
6. Venzor J, Lee WL, Huston DP. Urticarial vasculitis. Clin Rev Allergy Immunol. 2002;23(2): 201–16
7. Monroe EW. Urticarial vasculitis: an updated review. J Am Acad Dermatol. 1981;5(1):88–95
8. Jones RR, Bhogal B, Dash A, Schifferli J. Urticaria and vasculitis: a continuum of histological and immunopathological changes. Br J Dermatol. 1983;108(6):695–703
9. Sanchez NP, Winkelmann RK, Schroeter AL, Dicken CH. The clinical and histopathologic spectrums of urticarial vasculitis: study of forty cases. J Am Acad Dermatol. 1982;7(5):599–605
10. Berg RE, Kantor GR, Bergfeld WF. Urticarial vasculitis. Int J Dermatol. 1988;27(7):468–72
11. Davis MD, Daoud MS, Kirby B, Gibson LE, Rogers RS 3rd. Clinicopathologic correlation of hypocomplementemic and normocomplementemic urticarial vasculitis. J Am Acad Dermatol. 1998;38(6 Pt 1):899–905
12. Kano Y, Orihara M, Shiohara T. Cellular and molecular dynamics in exercise-induced urticarial vasculitis lesions. Arch Dermatol. 1998;134(1):62–7
13. Wisnieski JJ. Urticarial vasculitis. Curr Opin Rheumatol. 2000;12(1):24–31
14. Wisnieski JJ, Baer AN, Christensen J, Cupps TR, Flagg DN, Jones JV, et al Hypocomplementemic urticarial vasculitis syndrome. Clinical and serologic findings in 18 patients. Medicine (Baltimore) 1995;74(1):24–41
15. McDuffie FC, Sams WM Jr, Maldonado JE, Andreini PH, Conn DL, Samayoa EA. Hypocomplementemia with cutaneous vasculitis and arthritis. Possible immune complex syndrome. Mayo Clin Proc. 1973;48(5):340–8
16. Houser SL, Askenase PW, Palazzo E, Bloch KJ. Valvular heart disease in patients with hypocomplementemic urticarial vasculitis syndrome associated with Jaccoud's arthropathy. Cardiovasc Pathol. 2002;11(4):210–6
17. Callen JP, Kalbfleisch S. Urticarial vasculitis: a report of nine cases and review of the literature. Br J Dermatol. 1982;107(1):87–93
18. Kobayashi S, Nagase M, Hidaka S, Arai T, Ikegaya N, Hishida A, Honda N. Membranous nephropathy associated with hypocomplementemic urticarial vasculitis: report of two cases and a review of the literature. Nephron 1994;66(1):1–7
19. Schwartz HR, McDuffie FC, Black LF, Schroeter AL, Conn DL. Hypocomplementemic urticarial vasculitis: association with chronic obstructive pulmonary disease. Mayo Clin Proc. 1982;57(4):231–8
20. Soter NA. Urticarial vasculitis. In: Champion RH, Greaves MW, Kobza-Black A, Pye RJ, editors. The urticarias. Edinburgh: Churchill Livingstone; 1985. p. 141–8
21. Zeiss CR, Burch FX, Marder RJ, Furey NL, Schmid FR, Gewurz H. A hypocomplementemic vasculitic urticarial syndrome. Report of four new cases and definition of the disease. Am J Med. 1980;68(6):867–75
22. Eiser AR, Singh P, Shanies HM. Sustained dapsone-induced remission of hypocomplementemic urticarial vasculitis–a case report. Angiology 1997;48(11):1019–22
23. Borcea A, Greaves MW. Methotrexate-induced exacerbation of urticarial vasculitis: an unusual adverse reaction. Br J Dermatol. 2000;143(1):203–4

Angioedema

5.10

Elena Borzova and Clive E. H. Grattan

Core Messages

- Angioedema without weals is a distinct clinical pattern with different etiologies. It may require a management different from that of angioedema with weals.
- Histaminergic angioedema in chronic urticaria, allergic reactions, and physical urticarias develops rapidly and improves on epinephrine, corticosteroids, and antihistamines.
- In contrast, ACEI-associated angioedema, hereditary angioedema, and some cases of idiopathic angioedema are thought to be mediated by bradykinin; progress less rapidly; and respond poorly to epinephrine, steroids, and antihistamines.
- ACEI-induced angioedema may occur several years after the start of treatment. Patients of Afro-Carribean origin, those with hereditary or acquired angioedema, ACE inhibitor associated cough, and also immunocompromised cardiac and renal transplant patients are at increased risk of developing ACEI-induced angioedema.

Angioedema is defined by transient localized swellings of the deep reticular dermis, subcutaneous, or submucosal tissues. The potentially life-threatening nature of oropharyngeal and laryngeal swellings and an increasing rate of hospital admissions due to it over the last two decades [1] emphasize its importance. Nevertheless, delays in correct diagnosis of certain subtypes, including C1 esterase inhibitor deficiency and angiotensin converting enzyme inhibitor (ACEI)-induced angioedema, highlight the need for a better recognition to ensure optimal management.

E. Borzova (✉)
Department of Dermatology, Norfolk and Norwich University Hospital, Norwich NR4 7UY, UK
e-mail: elena.borzova@nnuh.nhs.uk

T. Zuberbier et al. (eds.), *Urticaria and Angioedema*,
DOI: 10.1007/978-3-540-79048-8_5.10, © Springer Verlag Berlin Heidelberg 2010

5.10.1 Classification of Angioedema

Angioedema may occur with or without weals. Angioedema with weals requires similar assessment and management to other presentations of urticaria [2], and therefore will not be discussed in this chapter. In contrast, angioedema without weals represents a distinct clinical pattern [3]. It is, nevertheless, a heterogeneous entity with several etio-pathophysiological subtypes sharing the same clinical manifestations. These subtypes can be defined by their causes and responsible mechanisms (Table 5.10.1).

Allergic angioedema is characterized by a close temporal relationship with exposure to the relevant allergen; requires prior sensitization; and recurs on reexposure to the same or cross-reacting allergens.

Nonsteroidal antiinflammatory drug (NSAID)-induced angioedema is thought to be caused by cyclo-oxygenase (COX) pathway inhibition with overproduction of cysteinyl leukotrienes. Angioedema may develop up to 24 h after exposure to the NSAID, but usually within 1–4 h [4]. Cross-reactions between NSAIDs are common; occur upon first exposure; and appear to be related to the potency of NSAID for inhibition of COX-1 isoenzyme. Aspirin, diclofenac, indomethacin, and ibuprofen are potent COX-1 inhibitors and thus often cross-react. In terms of in vitro inhibitory concentration (IC50) of NSAIDS for COX-1 enzyme, the potency of ibuprofen is four times as high as that of aspirin, while indomethacin (IC50 0.01 μM) appears to be about three times more potent than diclofenac (IC50 0.035 μM) and 1,000 times more than aspirin (IC50 10 μM). In contrast, weak inhibitors of COX-1 (IC50 > 1,000 μM), paracetamol, and the pyrazolones such as aminopyrine and phenacetin have less potential for cross-reactivity [5, 6].

ACEI-induced angioedema is the commonest cause of emergency hospital admissions with angioedema [7]. The prevalence of ACEI-induced angioedema in large clinical trials ranges from 0.4% of 4,645 patients treated with ramipril in the Heart Outcomes Prevention Evaluation (HOPE) study [8] to 0.68% of 12,557 patients who received enalapril in the recent OCTAVE study [9]. The incidence of ACEI associated angioedema is highest during the first month of therapy; however, some patients develop angioedema months, or even years, after initiation of the therapy [10]. Although angioedema has been a well-documented

Table 5.10.1 Angioedema without weals: etio-pathophysiological subtypes

Idiopathic angioedema
Allergic angioedema
NSAIDs-induced angioedema
ACE inhibitor-induced angioedema
Angioedema caused by C1 inhibitor deficiency
Hereditary angioedema
Acquired angioedema
Gleich syndrome
Angioedema induced by physical triggers
Vibratory angioedema
Exercise-induced angioedema

side effect of ACEI treatment since the mid-1980s and the early-onset association is well recognized by physicians, the late-onset presentation is often undiagnosed.

Hereditary angioedema (HAE) is an autosomal-dominant disorder caused by mutations in the C1 inhibitor (C1 inh) gene on chromosome 11 with a prevalence estimated at 1:50,000. C1 inhibitor is the only inhibitor of C1r and C1s; the major inhibitor of kallikrein and coagulation factor XII (although α2-macroglobulin can also inactivate these proteases) and can inhibit plasmin (although α2-antiplasmin is its main inhibitor), thereby playing a role in regulating the classical pathway of the complement cascade, kallikrein–kinin system, and possibly fibrinolysis. By inhibiting factor XIIa and factor XIa, C1 inh also controls the activation of the intrinsic coagulation pathway [11]. Therefore, C1 inh regulates the classical pathway of the complement, coagulation, fibrinolytic, and kallikrein–kinin systems. Its deficiency results in bradykinin overproduction leading to increased vascular permeability and angioedema [12].

There are two classical types of HAE: up to 85% of patients have HAE type I, in which the amount of active inhibitor is decreased to 30–50% of normal. In contrast, HAE type II is characterized by normal or even elevated levels of C1 inh, which lacks functional activity. Recently, a third type of HAE with an autosomal dominant inheritance has been described, which affects mostly women. It is characterized by a normal C1 inh level and function and appears to be oestrogen-dependent. Some authorities now prefer the term hereditary oestrogen-dependent angioedema to type III HAE to draw attention to the fact that it is not related to quantitative or qualitative changes in C1 inh. Mutations in the gene encoding the Factor of Hageman have recently been described in some families with the condition [13].

Angioedema with acquired C1 inh deficiency is very rare, being considerably less common than HAE and is frequently associated with B lymphocyte disorders ranging from monoclonal gammopathy of uncertain significance (MGUS) to B cell malignancies. The mechanisms responsible for acquired C1 inh deficiency are thought to be C1 inh consumption due to excessive complement activation or depletion of C1 inh by autoantibodies [14].

Angioedema can be triggered by a physical stimulus, such as vibratory angioedema. Delayed pressure urticaria swellings often have a deep component but do not conform to the typical presentation of angioedema. Exercise-induced angioedema is a rare type of angioedema, which may develop after any physical activity and can be a major disability to some patients.

There are two types of angioedema associated with eosinophilia: episodic and nonepisodic. Episodic angioedema with eosinophilia (Gleich's syndrome) is characterized by recurrent episodes of angioedema associated with weight gain (>18% of total body weight), fever, marked peripheral eosinophilia (>1,500/mm^3), an elevated IgM, no visceral involvement, and a favorable prognosis [15]. Gleich's syndrome is now regarded as one of the hypereosinophilic syndromes [16]. Nonepisodic angioedema with eosinophilia has been reported mostly in Japan and is diagnosed in patients, predominantly young women, with an attack of edema of bilateral upper or lower extremities associated with eosinophilia [15].

Idiopathic angioedema is diagnosed when no cause for angioedema can be identified. In a recent large patient series, idiopathic angioedema accounted for nearly 40% of patients presenting with angioedema without weals [17].

5.10.2 Pathophysiology of Angioedema

Several mediators are thought to be responsible for the increased vascular permeability resulting in clinical manifestations of angioedema. Clinical experience and recent research indicate that angioedema may be histaminergic or nonhistaminergic. These subtypes differ in their temporal evolution and response to treatment.

Histaminergic angioedema may be accompanied by weals, develops rapidly, and improves markedly with epinephrine, corticosteroids, and antihistamines. When untreated, most cases of histaminergic angioedema resolve within hours and no more than 2–3 days. By contrast, nonhistaminergic (bradykinin-mediated) angioedema progresses slowly, tends to subside within 3–5 days, and poorly responds to epinephrine, steroids, and antihistamines.

Angioedema associated with chronic urticaria, allergic reactions, or cold-induced urticaria is believed to be histamine-mediated, while bradykinin seems to be a crucial mediator of HAE and ACEI-induced angioedema. Of interest, idiopathic angioedema appears to be histaminergic in most cases but reveals nonhistaminergic features in about 14% of patients [17]. These cases of idiopathic nonhistaminergic angioedema may be well controlled by tranexamic acid [18]. Recognition of these pathophysiological patterns may have some clinical implications such as an expected response to treatment. However, the clinician should bear in mind a certain degree of oversimplification with this approach. For example, NSAIDs-induced angioedema may clinically be identical to histaminergic angioedema.

5.10.3 Clinical Features of Angioedema

Clinical manifestations of angioedema depend on its location: subcutaneous, intestinal, or laryngeal. Subcutaneous angioedema is nonpitting and nonpruritic, affecting the face, hands, feet, and genitalia most commonly but can involve any area of the body (Fig. 5.10.1). It can be disfiguring and immobilizing [19]. Patients with intestinal angioedema present with sudden onset, diffuse, and often severe colicky abdominal pain, which can be accompanied by nausea, vomiting, and watery diarrhea. On physical examination, they may have abdominal tenderness with no signs of peritonitis. Endoscopic examination reveals segmental mucosal edema without signs of inflammation. Computerized tomography scan features of intestinal angioedema include segmental bowel thickening and ascites. [20–22]. Swellings involving the tongue, pharynx, and larynx may result in airway compromise, which can be life-threatening [23]. Dyspnoea, dysphagia, and dysphonia are the clinical features of progressing laryngeal angioedema.

In addition, some clinical features can be characteristic for different angioedema subtypes. Thus, HAE attacks usually manifest in childhood or adolescence in 40% by the age of 5 and in 75% by the age of 12 [24]. They can be triggered by trauma, stress, and infections. In some patients, attacks are preceded by prodromal symptoms of a reticulate rash

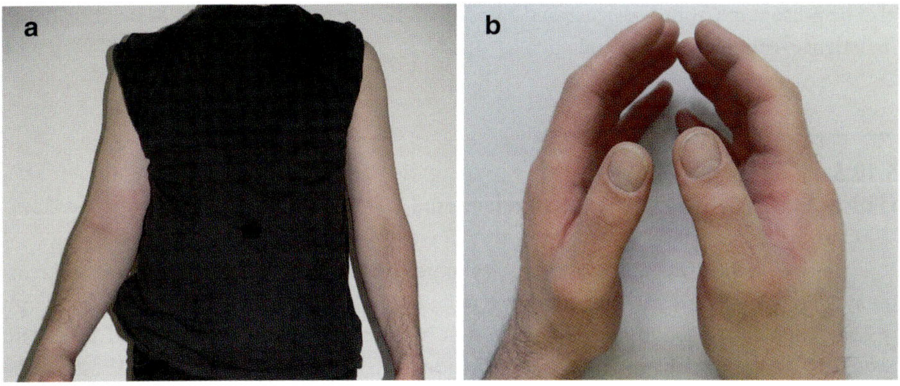

Fig. 5.10.1 Herideritary Angioedema in the arm of a patient (**a**); detail of hand (**b**) ©ECARF, used with permission

[25], irritability, headache, paraesthesia, and flu-like symptoms [26]. Female patients with HAE appear to have more attacks per year and more laryngeal symptoms [27]. Clinical features of ACEI-induced angioedema include its predilection to the lower face, tongue, and larynx. An increased risk of ACEI-induced angioedema has been reported in patients of Afro-Carribean origin, in those with hereditary or acquired angioedema, in those with ACE inhibitor associated cough [28], and also in immunocompromised cardiac and renal transplant patients [29]. Patients on ACEI may develop angioedema as a result of trauma during operations [23] and seem to be more prone to anaphylactic reactions to bee stings, venom immunotherapy [30], and during hemodialysis [31]. Nonallergic anaphylactic reactions during hemodialysis with negatively charged acrylonitrile membranes (for example, high-flux polyacrylonitrile AN69 membrane) in patients taking ACEI can be explained by bradykinin accumulation due to activation of the contact coagulation system by electronegatively charged surfaces, particularly under conditions of reduced bradykinin degradation by ACEI [32].

5.10.4 Differential Diagnosis of Angioedema

It is important to distinguish angioedema from other conditions resembling angioedema [33]. The onset and the duration of swelling as well as response to treatment usually give a clear indication of the differential diagnosis. Acute contact dermatitis can start with an angioedema-like swelling, particularly when the face is involved, before progressing to eczematous features and usually lasts for days or weeks. Cellulitis may manifest with local swelling accompanied by pain, redness, and fever. Persistent swellings can be diagnosed from the history, physical examination, laboratory evaluation, and biopsy. Melkersson–Rosenthal syndrome is characterized by persistent lip swelling associated with a fissured tongue (lingua plicata) and facial nerve palsy. Persistent lip swellings (cheilitis granulomatosa) may also be present in Crohn's disease and sarcoidosis. Dermatomyositis should be considered in patients with persistent eyelid edema.

5.10.5 Clinical Approach to a Patient with Angioedema

Recognition of the different angioedema subtypes is important to ensure appropriate treatment (Fig. 5.10.2). All patients with recurrent angioedema without weals should undergo investigation for C1 inhibitor deficiency, first by screening for C4 and then, if low, with tests for C1 inhibitor quantification and function [34]. In case of borderline test results, the C1 inhibitor function should be retested on fresh serum and then another method (colorimetric or C1s binding assays) if the result is still equivocal [35]. Allergic hypersensitivity as a cause for angioedema can be evaluated by a thorough history and allergy testing, when appropriate. Recurrent swellings in patients on ACEI should be assumed to be due to the drugs, which should be discontinued. Clinical experience suggests that the diagnosis of ACEI-induced angioedema is confirmed if recurrent angioedema attacks cease within approximately 1 month of ACEI withdrawal. If swelling attacks continue after the drug has been discontinued, the clinical situation should be regarded as unmasking other angioedema subtypes (HAE or idiopathic angioedema) by ACEI [36]. Angioedema induced by physical factors can be diagnosed by appropriate physical challenge tests. Episodic angioedema associated with persistent high blood eosinophilia should be suspicious for Gleich's syndrome. If no known causes can be identified, angioedema in these patients is considered to be idiopathic.

Emergency care for patients with angioedema depends on where it is and the presumed mechanism. HAE attacks of the oropharynx and bowel should be treated intravenously with C1 inhibitor concentrate [37]. Fresh frozen plasma can be an alternative in countries

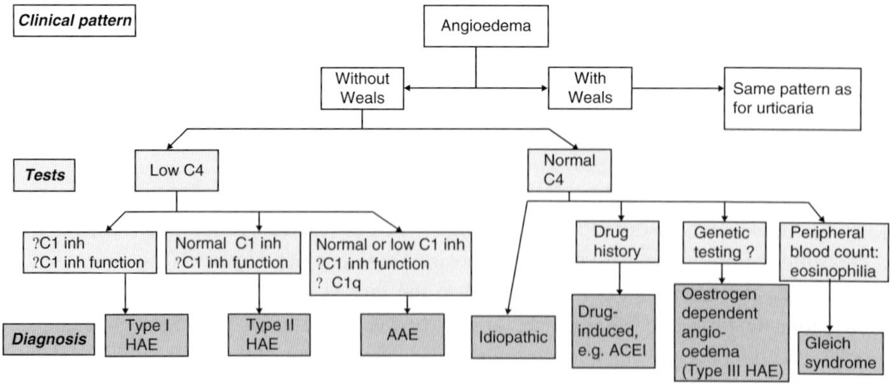

Fig. 5.10.2 Diagonistic algorithm for differential diagnosis of angioedema

where C1 inhibitor concentrate is not available. In other angioedema subtypes, intramuscular epinephrine injections (the dose depends on body weight) should be given in all cases of severe angioedema and repeated, if necessary after 10 min. Patients with laryngeal angioedema should be monitored closely and endotracheal intubation, tracheostomy, or cricothyroidotomy should be performed if essential [38]. Pain relief and fluid replacement are important in intestinal angioedema [39]. Parenteral antihistamines and steroids may be helpful in most cases of histaminergic angioedema.

Prophylaxis of angioedema should be tailored individually, based on angioedema severity and clinical subtypes of angioedema. Low-dose attenuated androgens are effective as prophylaxis for HAE patients but may be associated with significant toxicity (hepatitis, hepatoma, virilization, weight gain, and lipid profile changes) [34, 40]. Antifibrinolytic agents, ε-aminocaproic acid and tranexamic acid, can be used for HAE prophylaxis in patients for whom attenuated androgens are contraindicated, notably children and pregnant women [34, 40]. Potential side effects include muscle weakness, myalgia, and vascular thrombosis including the retina. Treatment with tranexamic acid may be effective for acquired angioedema and idiopathic nonhistaminergic angioedema [18]. Successful treatment of an underlying B-cell disorder should be beneficial for acquired angioedema [14]. Angiotensin II receptor antagonists should be used with caution in patients with ACEI-induced angioedema, since there have been a few reports of the persistence of angioedema [41]. ACEIs should be avoided in all patients with angioedema without weals, whatever the cause, but not necessarily in those with other presentations of urticaria. Episodic angioedema in Gleich's syndrome can be treated with long-term steroids or intravenous immunoglobulin therapy [15, 42]. All patients with recurrent angioedema should be encouraged to carry a MedicAlert bracelet and those with a history of severe tongue or throat angioedema should be offered self-administered epinephrine [43].

5.10.6
Recent Advances and Perspectives

Over the last 5 years, there have been important advances in our understanding of clinical, pathophysiological, and genetic aspects of angioedema.

Clinical advances encompass a better definition of angioedema subtypes and important changes in patient care. As a part of the PreHAEAT EU project, the European C1 inhibitor deficiency Working Group established the European HAE Register (http://www.haeregister.org) for collecting clinical and laboratory data on HAE patients. In March 2007, the first pooled data on 1,168 HAE patients from 10 European countries provided significant insights into the natural history of the disease [27]. Furthermore, recognition of the impact of recurrent angioedema on a patient's quality of life due to unpredictable, disfiguring, and potentially life-threatening angioedema attacks prompts a greater emphasis on self-administration therapy including a prescription of epinephrine syringes for patients with severe angioedema or home therapy with C1 inhibitor concentrate for HAE patients [44]. This can ensure greater security, reduced emotional distress, and better social functioning for these patients [45].

Significant progress has been made in our understanding of the pathophysiology of angioedema. Clinical research and experiments with C1 inhibitor knock-out mice provided evidence for bradykinin as a primary mediator of the increased vascular permeability in HAE [12], thereby providing new insight into therapeutic targets. A novel therapeutic agent targeting the kinin pathway, a kallikrein inhibitor DX-88 is under development and a bradykinin B2 receptor antagonist icatibant is now licensed for the emergency treatment of HAE patients and possibly for patients with other types of bradykinin-mediated angioedema in the near future.

More than 190 mutations of the C1 inhibitor gene have been registered in an online HAE mutation database (http://hae.biomembrane.hu) (on October 2007), thus yielding important knowledge on the genetic background of HAE. Remarkably, the first patient with homozygous C1 inhibitor gene mutations has been reported [46]. Genetic testing in HAE, when it becomes more widely available, can be particularly helpful for diagnosis in patients with no family history (up to 25% of all HAE patients) [47], with borderline complement test results [48], or possibly for revealing the Hageman factor gene mutations in patients with hereditary oestrogen-dependent angioedema [49]. Genetic tests may also enable the screening of family members at high risk and the prenatal diagnosis of HAE.

Furthermore, genetic technologies may modify the treatment interventions in patients with angioedema. Pharmacogenetic screening tests may allow us to identify patients at high risk for angioedema before commencing the treatment with ACEIs. This seems feasible on the strength of recent data reporting the C-2399A variant in XPNPEP2 gene encoding aminopeptidase P to be associated with a reduced activity of this enzyme and a higher incidence of ACEI-induced angioedema [50]. Advances in genetic technologies have the potential to affect the treatment modalities for HAE with a recombinant C1 inhibitor being developed for HAE [51] and also with a promise of the gene therapy [52] in the future.

5.10.7 Take Home Pearls

- All patients with recurrent angioedema without weals should have screening for C4 followed by tests for C1 inhibitor quantification and function if low.
- ACEI should be avoided in patients presenting with angioedema without weals.
- Swellings of the tongue, pharynx, and larynx may result in airway compromise, which can be life-threatening. HAE attacks of the oropharynx and bowel should be treated with C1 inhibitor concentrate. In other angioedema subtypes, severe laryngeal angioedema should be treated with intramuscular epinephrine.
- Patients with HAE and idiopathic angioedema often require prophylaxis. Treatment of an underlying B-cell disorder should be beneficial in acquired angioedema. Idiopathic angioedema without weals my respond to tranexamic acid.

References

1. Lin RY, Cannon AG, Teitel AD. Pattern of hospitalizations for angioedema in New York between 1990 and 2003. Ann Allergy Asthma Immunol. 2005;95(2):159–66
2. Zuberbier T, Bindslev-Jensen C, Canonica W, Grattan CE, Greaves MW, Henz BM, Kapp A, Kozel MM, Maurer M, Merk HF, Schafer T, Simon D, Vena GA, Wedi B. EAACI/GA2LEN/EDF. EAACI/GA2LEN/EDF guideline: definition, classification and diagnosis of urticaria. Allergy 2006;61(3):316–20
3. Grattan CE. The urticaria spectrum: recognition of clinical patterns can help management. Clin Exp Dermatol. 2004;29(3):217–21
4. Grattan CE. Aspirin sensitivity and urticaria. Clin Exp Dermatol. 2003;28(2):123–7
5. Sanchez-Borges M, Capriles-Hulett A, Caballero-Fonseca F. Hypersensitivity reactions to weak COX inhibitors. Allergy Clin Immunol Int. 2005;17:58–63
6. Woessner KM. Crossreacting drugs and chemicals. Clin Rev Allergy Immunol. 2003;24(2): 149–158
7. Kaplan AP, Greaves MW. Angioedema. J Am Acad Dermatol. 2005;53(3):373–88
8. Yusuf S, Sleight P, Pogue J, Bosch J, Davies R, Dagenais G. Effects of an angiotensin-converting-enzyme inhibitor, ramipril, on cardiovascular events in high-risk patients. The Heart Outcomes Prevention Evaluation Study Investigators. N Engl J Med. 2000;342(3):145–53. Erratum in: 2000;342(18):1376. N Engl J Med 2000;342(10):748
9. Kostis JB, Packer M, Black HR, Schmieder R, Henry D, Levy E. Omapatrilat and enalapril in patients with hypertension: the Omapatrilat Cardiovascular Treatment vs. Enalapril (OCTAVE) trial. Am J Hypertens. 2004;17(2):103–11
10. Byrd JB, Adam A, Brown NJ. Angiotensin-converting enzyme inhibitor-associated angioedema. Immunol Allergy Clin North Am. 2006;26(4):725–37
11. Davis AE III. Mechanism of angioedema in first complement component inhibitor deficiency. Immunol Allergy Clin North Am. 2006;26(4):633–51
12. Davis AE III. The pathophysiology of hereditary angioedema. Clin Immunol. 2005;114(1): 3–9
13. Bork K. Hereditary angioedema with normal C1 inhibitor activity including hereditary angioedema with coagulation factor XII gene mutations. Immunol Allergy Clin North Am. 2006; 26(4):709–24
14. Zingale LC, Castelli R, Zanichelli A, Cicardi M. Acquired deficiency of the inhibitor of the first complement component: presentation, diagnosis, course, and conventional management. Immunol Allergy Clin North Am. 2006;26(4):669–90
15. Banerji A, Weller PF, Sheikh J. Cytokine-associated angioedema syndromes including episodic angioedema with eosinophilia (Gleich's Syndrome). Immunol Allergy Clin North Am. 2006; 26(4):769–81
16. Klion AD, Bochner BS, Gleich GJ, Nutman TB, Rothenberg ME, Simon HU, Wechsler ME, Weller PF; The Hypereosinophilic Syndromes Working Group. Approaches to the treatment of hypereosinophilic syndromes: a workshop summary report. J Allergy Clin Immunol. 2006;117(6):1292–302
17. Zingale LC, Beltrami L, Zanichelli A, Maggioni L, Pappalardo E, Cicardi B, Cicardi M. Angioedema without urticaria: a large clinical survey. CMAJ. 2006;175(9):1065–70
18. Cicardi M, Bergamaschini L, Zingale LC, Gioffre D, Agostoni A. Idiopathic nonhistaminergic angioedema. Am J Med. 1999;106(6):650–4
19. Bracho FA Hereditary angioedema. Curr Opin Hematol. 2005;12(6):493–8
20. Koruth JS, Eckardt AJ, Levey JM. Hereditary angioedema involving the colon: endoscopic appearance and review of GI manifestations. Gastrointest Endosc. 2005;61(7):907–11
21. Marmery H, Mirvis SE. Angiotensin-converting enzyme inhibitor-induced visceral angioedema. Clin Radiol. 2006;61(11):979–82

22. Schmidt TD, McGrath KM. Angiotensin-converting enzyme inhibitor angioedema of the intestine: a case report and review of the literature. Am J Med Sci. 2002;324(2):106–8
23. Sarkar P, Nicholson G, Hall G. Brief review: angiotensin converting enzyme inhibitors and angioedema: anesthetic implications. Can J Anaesth. 2006;53(10):994–1003
24. Fay A, Abinun M. Current management of hereditary angio-oedema (C'1 esterase inhibitor deficiency). J Clin Pathol. 2002;55(4):266–70
25. Williamson DW. Reticulate erythema – a prodrome in hereditary angio-oedema. Br J Derm 1979;1011:549–552
26. Gibbs JG, Craig TJ. Prodromal symptoms before exacerbations of hereditary angioedema. J Allergy Clin Immunol. 2007;119(1):S278
27. Zingale LC, Bork K, Farkas H, Bygum A, Bouillet L, Caballero T, Longhurst H, Waage Nielsen E, Bilo B, Bucher C, Perricone R, Cicardi M. The European register of hereditary angioedema: experience and preliminary results. J Allergy Clin Immunol 2007;119(1): S276
28. Morimoto T, Gandhi TK, Fiskio JM, Seger AC, So JW, Cook EF, Fukui T, Bates DW. An evaluation of risk factors for adverse drug events associated with angiotensin-converting enzyme inhibitors. J Eval Clin Pract. 2004;10(4):499–509
29. Abbosh J, Anderson JA, Levine AB, Kupin WL. Angiotensin converting enzyme inhibitor-induced angioedema more prevalent in transplant patients. Ann Allergy Asthma Immunol. 1999;82(5):473–6
30. Kemp SF, Lieberman P. Inhibitors of angiotensin ii: potential hazards for patients at risk for anaphylaxis? Ann Allergy Asthma Immunol. 1997;78(6):527–529
31. Kammerl MC, Schaefer RM, Schweda F, Schreiber M, Riegger GA, Kramer BK. Extracorporal therapy with AN69 membranes in combination with ACE inhibition causing severe anaphylactoid reactions: still a current problem? Clin Nephrol. 2000;53(6):486–8
32. Ebo DG, Bosmans JL, Couttenye MM, Stevens WJ. Haemodialysis-associated anaphylactic and anaphylactoid reactions. Allergy 2006;61:211–220
33. Weldon D. Differential diagnosis of angioedema. Immunol Allergy Clin North Am. 2006; 26(4):603–13
34. Gompels MM, Lock RJ, Abinun M, Bethune CA, Davies G, Grattan C, Fay AC, Longhurst HJ, Morrison L, Price A, Price M, Watters D. C1 inhibitor deficiency: consensus document. Clin Exp Immunol. 2005;139(3):379–94
35. Gompels MM, Lock RJ. Laboratory testing for C1 inhibitor deficiency: a comparison of two approaches to C1 inhibitor function. Ann Clin Biochem. 2007;44(Pt 1):75–8
36. Ricketti AJ, Cleri DJ, Ramos-Bonner LS, Vernaleo JR. Hereditary angioedema presenting in late middle age after angiotensin-converting enzyme inhibitor treatment. Ann Allergy Asthma Immunol. 2007;98(4):397–401
37. Longhurst HJ. Emergency treatment of acute attacks in hereditary angioedema due to C1 inhibitor deficiency: what is the evidence? Int J Clin Pract. 2005;59(5):594–9
38. Chiu AG, Newkirk KA, Davidson BJ, Burningham AR, Krowiak EJ, Deeb ZE. Angiotensin-converting enzyme inhibitor-induced angioedema: a multicenter review and an algorithm for airway management. Ann Otol Rhinol Laryngol. 2001;110(9):834–40
39. Oudit G, Girgrah N, Allard J. ACE inhibitor-induced angioedema of the intestine: case report, incidence, pathophysiology, diagnosis and management. Can J Gastroenterol. 2001;15(12): 827–32
40. Bowen T, Cicardi M, Farkas H, Bork K, Kreuz W, Zingale L, Varga L, Martinez-Saguer I, Aygoren-Pursun E, Binkley K, Zuraw B, Davis A III, Hebert J, Ritchie B, Burnham J, Castaldo A, Menendez A, Nagy I, Harmat G, Bucher C, Lacuesta G, Issekutz A, Warrington R, Yang W, Dean J, Kanani A, Stark D, McCusker C, Wagner E, Rivard GE, Leith E, Tsai E, MacSween M, Lyanga J, Serushago B, Leznoff A, Waserman S, de Serres J. Canadian 2003 international consensus algorithm for the diagnosis, therapy, and management of hereditary angioedema. J Allergy Clin Immunol. 2004;114(3):629–37

41. Sica DA, Black HR. Current concepts of pharmacotherapy in hypertension: ACE inhibitor-related angioedema: can angiotensin-receptor blockers be safely used? J Clin Hypertens (Greenwich). 2002;4(5):375–80
42. Orson FM. Intravenous immunoglobulin therapy suppresses manifestations of the angioedema with hypereosinophilia syndrome. Am J Med Sci. 2003;326(2):94–7
43. Sabroe RA, Glendinning AK, Sabroe I, Lawlor F, Kobza Black A. An audit of the use of self-administered adrenaline syringes in patients with angio-oedema. Br J Dermatol. 2002;146(4): 615–20
44. Longhurst HJ, Carr S, Khair K. C1-inhibitor concentrate home therapy for hereditary angioedema: a viable, effective treatment option. Clin Exp Immunol. 2007;147(1):11–7
45. Levi M, Choi G, Picavet C, Hack CE. Self-administration of C1-inhibitor concentrate in patients with hereditary or acquired angioedema caused by C1-inhibitor deficiency. J Allergy Clin Immunol. 2006;117(4):904–8
46. Blanch A, Roche O, Urrutia I, Gamboa P, Fontan G, Lopez-Trascasa M. First case of homozygous C1 inhibitor deficiency. J Allergy Clin Immunol. 2006;118(6):1330–5
47. Sachse MM, Khachemoune A, Guldbakke KK, Kirschfink M. Hereditary angioedema. J Drugs Dermatol. 2006;5(9):848–52
48. Weiler CR, van Dellen RG. Genetic test indications and interpretations in patients with hereditary angioedema. Mayo Clin Proc. 2006;81(7):958–72
49. Dewald G, Bork K. Missense mutations in the coagulation factor XII (Hageman factor) gene in hereditary angioedema with normal C1 inhibitor. Biochem Biophys Res Commun. 2006;343(4):1286–9
50. Nikpoor B, Duan QL, Rouleau GA. Acute adverse reactions associated with angiotensin-converting enzyme inhibitors: genetic factors and therapeutic implications. Expert Opin Pharmacother. 2005;6(11):1851–6
51. Zuraw BL. Novel therapies for hereditary angioedema. Immunol Allergy Clin North Am. 2006;26(4):691–708
52. Chinen J, Puck JM. Successes and risks of gene therapy in primary immunodeficiencies. J Allergy Clin Immunol. 2004;113(4):595–603

Therapy of Urticaria

6

Bettina Wedi

Core Messages

- The different urticaria subtypes are common skin diseases persisting often for years with multifactorial triggering factors and greatly reduced quality of life as well as occupational disability.
- Therapy can be problematic and is not standardised. Regarding the long duration of this annoying skin disease, every attempt should be made to identify and avoid specific or unspecific triggering factors. The treatment goal is to maximise the quality of life, to maintain vigilance and ability to work or to attend school and to minimise drug-related side effects.
- Besides antihistamines and the eradication or avoidance of identified triggering factors, many drugs, most of which are not licensed for urticaria, are administered.
- The highest grade of recommendation (GoR) according to the criteria of evidence-based medicine can only be given for second-generation H1 antihistamines. They should be administered in an adequate dose, up to fourfold the normal dose while considering potential side effects.
- The data on treatment alternatives are totally insufficient. Good evidence exists in severely affected patients for cyclosporin A. Subgroups might benefit from addition of leukotrienes antagonists. Chloroquine and dapsone may be worthy of further investigation within randomised controlled trials.
- The risk–benefit profile of each alternative (off-label use) to second-generation H1 antihistamines should be carefully considered before treatment. This applies especially to immunosuppressive agents.

B. Wedi
Department of Dermatology and Allergology, Hannover Medical University, Ricklinger Strasse 5, 30449 Hannover, Germany
e-mail: wedi.bettina@mh-hannover.de

T. Zuberbier et al. (eds.), *Urticaria and Angioedema*,
DOI: 10.1007/978-3-540-79048-8_6, © Springer Verlag Berlin Heidelberg 2010

The clinical pictures of urticaria are of heterogeneous aetiology and therefore subclassified into distinct groups, which can coexist: spontaneous urticaria, physical urticaria and special types. To optimise urticaria treatment, the first strategy should be to correctly classify the respective urticaria subtype. The treatment goal is to maximise the quality of life and ability to work or to attend school and to minimise drug-related side effects. This is of particular importance regarding the long year duration of many urticaria subtypes. Relevant outcomes of treatment trials include pruritus, weal size, number and frequency, loss of awakening, overall physician and patient assessment and permanent remission of disease.

This chapter is based on the results of two recent publications evaluating randomised controlled trials (RCTs) of urticaria therapy (until October 2004) according to the criteria of evidence-based medicine [1, 2]. Details of the individual studies, inclusion and exclusion criteria as well as the cited literature are available in the publications [1, 2], if not otherwise cited. Additionally, this review includes at least the RCTs published until December 2006 [3–7] and also interesting treatment approaches. In the text, the respective GoR according to the criteria of evidence-based medicine of the Scottish Intercollegiate Guidelines Network (SIGN; www.sign.ac.uk, GoR A to D, whereas A represents best evidence) is given in parentheses. Table 6.1 summarises the recommended therapeutic approaches.

6.1 General Treatment Advice for All Urticaria Subtypes

Every attempt should be made to find an underlying aetiology in each patient, because the identification and elimination of causal factors represent the best therapeutic approach. Co-existing trigger factors may also require treatment.

Every identified triggering factor should be avoided or adequately treated (GoR D). Principally, the intake of non-steroidal anti-inflammatory drugs (NSAID), particularly of acetylsalicylic acid (ASA), should be avoided (GoR D). Often, regular intake of these drugs is not reported. ASA exacerbates urticaria symptoms in 20–30% of cases. Usually, paracetamol (acetaminophen) is tolerated. Other mast cell activating drugs are morphine, codeine, muscle relaxants, polymyxin and dextran.

In the case of recurrent angio-oedema (with or without wealing), ACE-inhibitors and angiotensin II receptor antagonists (sartans) should not be given (GoR D).

Moreover, alcohol, stress and overheating may aggravate urticaria (GoR D). Detailed explanation and information, patient diaries and a good physician–patient relationship are helpful in the management.

6.2 Evidence-Based Treatment of Spontaneous Urticaria

6.2.1 Spontaneous Acute Urticaria

Spontaneous acute urticaria can be of allergic or non-allergic nature. However, symptomatic treatment of the clinical manifestation does not differ. Medical supervision (inpatient

Table 6.1 Evidence-based treatment of urticaria subtypes. GoR, grade of recommendation (according to criteria of the Scottish Intercollegiate Guidelines Network, http://www.sign.ac.uk)

Urticaria subtype		Recommendation
All subtypes		*GoR D* Elimination of causal factors Avoid intake of NSAID (ASA!) or mast cell activating drugs Avoid ACE-inhibitors, sartans (in case of recurrent angio-oedema) Avoid overheating, stress, alcohol Antipruritic, cooling lotions Provide with rescue medication (in case of severe angio-oedema, anaphylaxis)
spontaneous urticaria	Acute	*GoR D* Low sedating H1-AH, up to fourfold daily Glucocorticosteroids orally or i.v. (acute severe reactions) Epinephrine (anaphylaxis)
	Chronic	*GoR A* Daily standard dose of low sedating H1-AH *GoR B* Combination of low sedating H1-AH with cyclosporine A (2.5–5 mg/kg/day) *GoR C* Up to fourfold dose of low sedating H1-AH daily Eradication of Helicobacter pylori infection *GoR D* Causal treatment Eradication of other infections Standardised pseudoallergen-low diet Thyroid hormones *Combination of low sedating H1-AH with* First choice Leukotrienes antagonists Second choice Glucocorticosteroids (oral short course) Chloroquine Dapsone Third choice (alphabetic order) Autologous whole blood injections (in ASST+ patients.), cox-2 inhibitors, cyclophosphamide, doxepine, interferon, Ketotifen, methotrexate, mycophenolate mofetil, nifedipine, oxatomide, Stanazolol, sulphasalazine, Tacrolimus, terbutaline, theophylline, Warfarin, plasmapheresis, intravenous immunoglobulins
Physical urticaria	Dermographic	*GoR D* Low sedating H1-AH, up to fourfold daily KETOTIFEN

(*continued*)

Table 6.1 (continued)

Urticaria subtype		Recommendation
	cold	*GoR B* Low sedating H1-AH *GoR D* Low sedating H1-AH, up to fourfold daily *Combination with* First choice Penicillin i.m. or p.o. Doxycycline or tetracycline p.o. Second choice Cyproheptadine, Ketotifen, Montelukast, omalizumab (anti-IgE)
	Delayed pressure	*GoR D* Low sedating H1-AH, up to fourfold daily *Combination with (alphabetic)* Clobetasol prop. 0.5% ointment, dapsone, glucocorticosteroids (up to 40 mg/day), Ketotifen plus nimesulide, methotrexate, montelukast, sulphaasalazine
	Localised heat	*GoR D* Skin hardening to heat Chloroquine
	Solar	*GoR D* Low sedating H1-AH Cyclosporine A, Chloroquine, photo hardening of the skin, plasmapheresis, photopheresis, plasma exchange, intravenous immunoglobulins
	Vibratory	*GoR D* Avoidance of vibrating forces
Special types	Cholinergic	*GoR D* Low sedating H1-AH, up to fourfold daily *Combination with* Danazol, Ketotifen, scopolamine butylbromide
	Aquagenic	*GoR D* Low sedating H1-AH, up to fourfold daily

care) is recommended in case of dyspnea, hypotension and generalised severe urticaria. Causal treatment includes stopping of culprit drug intake, removing insect stinger and prescription of antibiotics in bacterial infections.

With respect to acute urticaria, only four low-quality RCTs have been published investigating low-sedating H1 antihistamines or short courses of corticosteroids [2].

Symptomatic treatment consists of low-sedating H1-antihistamines (GoR D) up to fourfold daily (consider potential side effects when increasing the dose!) (GoR D). If favoured, local treatment with antipruritic and cooling lotions may be added (GoR D). In severe cases (associated severe angio-oedema), often additional administration of glucocorticosteroids up to 100–250 mg prednisolone (i.v.) and H1-antihistamine (i.v.) are needed (GoR D), may be repeatedly (GoR D). In progressive cases, anaphylactic shock treatment including proper administration of epinephrine is mandatory (GoR D). Most cases improve promptly after (i.v.) treatment with antihistamines and glucocorticosteroids. However, symptoms may re-occur several hours later (in most patients total symptoms persist for less than 2 weeks). Therefore, outpatients should take low-sedating antihistamines in adequate doses (up to fourfold) for 1–2 weeks (GoR D) and should be provided with a rescue medication (GoR D), e.g., drinkable corticosteroid, for severe symptoms. The therapeutic use of H2 antihistamines in acute urticaria is far from being clear. Topical antihistamines should be avoided due to their limited effect and sensitising potential.

There is no prognostic factor identifying patients at risk for progression to chronic urticaria (less than 1%), but it is discussed that adequate treatment of acute urticaria is able to inhibit progression to chronic urticaria.

6.2.2 Spontaneous Chronic Urticaria

Chronic urticaria usually persists for at least 3–5 years. In those 40% lasting more than 6 months, chronic urticaria is still present 10 years later and in 20%, even after 20 years. The best therapeutic approach is to eliminate a causal triggering factor. Standardised diagnostic procedures have been published elsewhere [8, 9].

6.2.2.1 Treatment of Persistent Infections

A systematic review of published studies on chronic urticaria and Helicobacter pylori infection showed that remission of urticaria is significantly more likely following eradication [10] (GoR C). Numerous treatment strategies exist, but even the best (French or Italian triple therapy) fail in about 20% of cases. Therefore, success of therapy must be established, for example, by means of a breath test or renewed gastroscopy 4–6 weeks after treatment.

Moreover, other persistent, chronic, usually subclinical infections with, for example, streptococci, staphylococci or yersinia, may be responsible (GoR D) [11, 12]. For streptococci and staphylococci, oral cephalosporines (e.g., cefuroxime axetil 500 mg b.i.d. for 12 days), for persistent yersiniosis (with elevated IgA and corresponding bands in the immunoblot) a fluoroquinolone (e.g., ciprofloxacin 500 mg b.i.d. for 10 days) or the combination of trimethoprim and sulphamethoxazole (800/160 mg b.i.d. for 10 days) are a good choice. No RCTs exist for treatment of these infections regarding the outcome of chronic urticaria [11].

6.2.2.2 Diet

IgE-mediated sensitisations to food may play a role in spontaneous acute urticaria, particularly in atopic patients. However, in chronic urticaria IgE-mediated food allergy is very rare. Nevertheless, some patients may be triggered by food additives, and possibly by biogenic amines via non-allergic so far undetermined mechanisms [13]. Before a therapeutic diet

(GoR D) is recommended, first a standardised pseudoallergen-low diet [14] followed by blinded and placebo-controlled oral provocation tests should have proven exacerbation of the spontaneous urticaria [15].

6.2.2.3 Non-Sedating H1 Antihistamines

Long-acting low-sedating antihistamines are the mainstay of symptomatic treatment and can be given the highest GoR according to the criteria of evidence-based medicine (GoR A). They reduce itch, weal duration and numbers and increase the quality of life. The current European Guideline recommends an increased dose up to fourfold the normal dose while considering the side effects (GoR C). In the meantime, off-label doses of up to threefold have been described to be effective and safe [16].

Owing to the long-term duration of the disease, low-sedating H1-antihistamines are preferred, particularly when increased dosage is needed. H1-antihistamines demonstrating high-quality evidence in chronic urticaria treatment include: azelastine, cetirizine, desloratadine, ebastine, fexofenadine, levocetirizine, loratadine and mizolastine (alphabetical order). Management is better achieved by taking antihistamines regularly, not just when needed.

Antihistamines are safe but potential side effects such as impairment of performance, sedation, interaction with CYP450 enzymes (for drugs metabolised via CYP450, see for example, http://medicine.iupui.edu/flockhart/table.htm), liver, cardiac side effects and nephrotoxicity should be considered for the respective choice. It is best to avoid all antihistamines in pregnancy, although teratogenic effects have not been proven. Flawless studies investigating alternatives in chronic urticaria are rare. Glucocorticosteroids (30–40 mg of prednisone per day) should only be used after a trial of maximal dose of antihistamines. Moreover, replacement of one H1-antihistamine with another should be tried because of individual differences in responsiveness.

6.2.2.4 H2-Antihistamines

The choice of a combination of an H1-antihistamine with an H2-antihistamine is not justified nowadays [1, 2]. The questionable synergism between H1 and H2 antagonists is probably due to a pharmacokinetic effect, i.e., the H2 blockers cause increased plasma levels of the H1 antihistamine [17]. This effect could not be demonstrated for the co-administration of cimetidine with modern H1 antihistamines such as cetirizine and ebastine. RCTs of a combination of H2 blockers and non-sedating H1 antihistamines have not been published.

6.2.2.5 Glucocorticosteroids

RCTs of the efficacy of glucocorticosteroids in chronic urticaria have not been published. There is consensus that glucocorticosteroids should only be used with caution, for example, to achieve short-term control of symptoms in acute exacerbations (GoR D). Side effects prohibit long-term use in high dosage. In isolated cases, especially in pressure-induced weals, low-dose steroids can be helpful (GoR D).

Restraint should be used in prescribing corticosteroids in diabetes, glaucoma, osteoporosis, gastrointestinal ulcers and obesity.

6.2.2.6 Leukotriene Antagonists

Data from published RCTs with different antileukotrienes are contradictory and difficult to compare. These drugs appear to be effective in certain sub-groups, for example, patients with a positive autologous serum test and/or intolerance of aspirin and/or food additives (GoR D) [1, 2, 18]. On the basis of the existing studies, it is impossible to determine whether monotherapy is equally effective to a combination with non-sedating H1-antihistamine. Our personal experience (in Germany, only Montelukast is licensed) is that monotherapy is ineffective.

6.2.2.7 Cyclosporin A

From an evidence-based viewpoint, the existing data suggest that the only useful, well-studied alternative for severely affected patients is cyclosporin A in combination with non-sedating H1-antihistamines. In 2006, a 16-week RCT confirmed the outcome of a prior well-done study [19] demonstrating the usefulness of cyclosporin A in antihistamine-resistant chronic urticaria (GoR B) [6]. Both studies used background therapy with cetirizine. Including uncontrolled trials and case series, different treatment strategies have been used; cyclosporin A 2.5 to 5 mg/kg/day or 5 mg/kg/day progressively reduced to 3 mg/kg/day. It remains unclear whether only subgroups, e.g., with a positive autologous serum test, profit from cyclosporin and whether long-term success can be achieved even after discontinuation.

Before administering cyclosporin A, a careful benefit–risk analysis should be undertaken owing to the serious potential side effects. Blood pressure, BUN, creatinine and serum lipids should be checked regularly. Cyclosporine is contraindicated when there is a history of malignancy or impaired renal function.

6.2.2.8 Thyroid Hormones

A strong association between chronic urticaria and thyroid autoimmunity has been demonstrated. A subset of patients with associated autoimmune thyroiditis may respond to the administration of thyroxine. A controlled trial is lacking (GoR D) [20].

6.2.2.9
Other Therapeutic Options

Several drugs have been used in treating chronic urticaria not responding to antihistamines. Most have been prescribed in combination with antihistamines. Using evidence-based criteria, only the lowest GoR D can be assigned to the following options: antidepressants (doxepin), mast cell stabilisers (oxatomide, ketotifen), calcium channel blockers (nifedipine) and sympathomimetics (terbutaline), warfarin and stanozolol. In light of high rates of side effects and limited benefit, these drugs cannot be recommended. Recent controlled studies found a benefit of autologous whole blood injections in autologous serum skin test positive patients (statistically not significant vs. placebo) [5] and of theophylline [3].

Evidence is based on case reports, case series or uncontrolled trials for drugs such as chloroquine, dapsone, sulphasalazine, tacrolimus, methotrexate, cyclophosphamide, mycophenolate mofetil [21], interferon and cox-2 inhibitors as well as for plasmapheresis and intravenous immunoglobulin infusions.

6.3
Evidence-Based Treatment of Physical Urticaria

Physical urticaria is a distinct group that is caused by external physical stimulus. Neither the pathomechanisms have been clarified, nor sufficient data are available to recommend treatment schedules based on an evidence-based view.

Dermographic urticaria is the most frequent subtype of physical urticaria and develops within a few minutes after mechanical shearing forces and presents with intensely itching weals, for example, after writing on the skin.

Treatment is similar to chronic urticaria with low-sedating H1-antihistamines given regularly and at adequate dose (up to fourfold the normal dose) (GoR D). Additional low evidence exists for Ketotifen (GoR D). Dermographic urticaria is distressing but not life-threatening.

Sustained vertical pressure is the eliciting factor of delayed deep, painful swellings in *delayed pressure urticaria*. Delayed pressure urticaria is more common in middle-aged males and persists for an average of 6–9 years, often resulting in disability to work. It may be associated with chronic urticaria.

Delayed pressure urticaria responds poorly to antihistamines, even in increased doses. Nevertheless, they represent the mainstay of treatment (GoR D). Some patients are well controlled by additional corticosteroids (e.g. 40–20 mg prednisone; GoR D), others by treatment with dapsone (100–150 mg/day; GoR D). Other low-evidence alternatives are methotrexate (15 mg/week; GoR D), montelukast, ketotifen plus nimesulide, sulphasalazine or topical clobetasol prop. 0.5% ointment (all GoR D).

Cold bodies or cold water, also cold air and cold food/drinks can provoke *cold urticaria* and angio-oedema within minutes. Mainly young adults are affected with an average duration of 5 years. It may coexist with cholinergic urticaria.

Identified infectious diseases such as syphilis, borreliosis, hepatitis, infectious mononucleosis and HIV infections should be treated adequately (GoR D). Low-sedating H1 antihistamines are the first line in treatment (GoR B). In idiopathic cases, antibiotic treatment (e.g., with doxycycline or penicillin, i.m. or p.o.) is worth trying (GoR D). Other low-evidence alternatives (all GoR D) are cyproheptadine, ketotifen and montelukast. A recent case report demonstrated remission after anti-IgE [22] (GoR D).

Localised heat urticaria is a rare phenomenon that is developed by direct contact with a warm object such as air or water (38°C to more than 50°C). Evidence-based treatment is not available. Skin hardening to heat or chloroquine may be tried (GoR D).

Solar urticaria to wavelengths ranging from 280 to 760 nm (mostly UV-light) is rare. Women in their third or forth decade of life are predominantly affected. Treatment can be frustrating. Low-sedating H1 antihistamines are the first line of treatment (GoR D). Photohardening of the skin may be effective (GoR D). Other low-evidence possibilities include plasmapheresis, cyclosporin A, photopheresis, plasma exchange, and intravenous immunoglobulins or chloroquine (all GoR D).

Very rarely strong vibrating forces (e.g., pneumatic hammer) result in *vibratory urticaria and/or angio-oedema*. Avoidance of vibrating forces is the treatment of choice.

6.4 Evidence-Based Treatment of Special Urticaria Subtypes

Cholinergic urticaria, common in young adults, is caused by a short increase in body temperature, e.g., by physical exercise, passive warmth (hot bath) or emotional stress. It is difficult to achieve exercise tolerance. Low-sedating H1-antihistamines (in increased dose) regularly or 1 h before characteristic triggering situations are the mainstay of treatment (GoR D). Nevertheless, they often fail. Ketotifen may be an optional medication (GoR D). Efficient treatment with Danazol has been described in single cases (GoR D), but adverse effects have to be considered.

Aquagenic urticaria is very rare. Contact to water of any temperature liberates a water-soluble allergen from the stratum corneum that diffuses into the dermis. In most cases, prophylactic treatment with low-sedating H1 antihistamines is sufficient (GoR D).

6.5 Take Home Pearls

- The clinical pictures of urticaria are of heterogeneous aetiology and subclassified into distinct groups, which can co-exist
- The treatment goal is to maximise the quality of life, to maintain vigilance and ability to work or to attend school and to minimise drug-related side effects
- Regarding the long duration of this annoying skin disease, every attempt should be made to identify and avoid triggering factors (e.g., infections or intake of pseudoallergens)

- For symptomatic treatment, best evidence exists for second-generation H1-antihistamines. These are the only drugs officially approved for treating urticaria
- First-line treatment consists of second-generation H1 antihistamines given regularly and in adequate dose
- Second-generation H1 antihistamines have a better therapeutic index and improved pharmacodynamic properties compared to their older counterparts
- Evidence for alternative treatment options is low and depends on the urticaria subtype
- Subgroups (i.e., with positive ASST, and/or intolerance to aspirin/food additives) might benefit from addition of leukotrienes antagonists
- Severely affected patients may be treated with cyclosporine A
- Chloroquine and dapsone may be worthy of further investigation within randomised controlled trials

References

1. Wedi B, Kapp A Chronic urticaria: assessment of current treatment. Exp Rev Clin Immunol. 2005;1:459–73
2. Zuberbier T, Bindslev-Jensen C, Canonica W, et al EAACI/GALEN/EDF guideline: management of urticaria. Allergy 2006;61:321–31
3. Kalogeromitros D, Kempuraj D, Katsarou-Katsari A, et al Theophylline as 'add-on' therapy to cetirizine in patients with chronic idiopathic urticaria. A randomized, double-blind, placebo-controlled pilot study. Int Arch Allergy Immunol. 2006;139:258–64
4. Nettis E, Colanardi MC, Soccio AL, et al Desloratadine in combination with montelukast suppresses the dermographometer challenge test papule, and is effective in the treatment of delayed pressure urticaria: a randomized, double-blind, placebo-controlled study. Br J Dermatol. 2006;155:1279–82
5. Staubach P, Onnen K, Vonend A, et al Autologous whole blood injections to patients with chronic urticaria and a positive autologous serum skin test: a placebo-controlled trial. Dermatology 2006;212:150–9
6. Vena GA, Cassano N, Colombo D, et al Cyclosporine in chronic idiopathic urticaria: a double-blind, randomized, placebo-controlled trial. J Am Acad Dermatol. 2006;55:705–9
7. Vena GA, Cassano N, D'Argento V, et al Clobetasol propionate 0.05% in a novel foam formulation is safe and effective in the short-term treatment of patients with delayed pressure urticaria: a randomized, double-blind, placebo-controlled trial. Br J Dermatol. 2006;154:353–6
8. Wedi B, Kapp A. [Diagnostics of urticaria]. Allergo J. 2006;15:205–10
9. Zuberbier T, Bindslev-Jensen C, Canonica W, et al EAACI/GALEN/EDF guideline: definition, classification and diagnosis of urticaria. Allergy 2006;61:316–20
10. Federman DG, Kirsner RS, Moriarty JP, et al The effect of antibiotic therapy for patients infected with *Helicobacter pylori* who have chronic urticaria. J Am Acad Dermatol. 2003;49:861–4
11. Wedi B, Raap U, Kapp A. Chronic urticaria and infections. Curr Opin Allergy Clin Immunol. 2004;4:387–96
12. Wedi B, Wagner S, Werfel T, et al Prevalence of *Helicobacter pylori*-associated gastritis in chronic urticaria. Int Arch Allergy Immunol. 1998;116:288–294
13. Wedi B, Kapp A. [Current position of the role of allergic and non-allergic food hypersensitivity in urticaria]. Hautarzt 2006;57:101–7
14. Zuberbier T, Chantraine-Hess S, Hartmann K, et al Pseudoallergen-free diet in the treatment of chronic urticaria. A prospective study. Acta Derm Venereol. 1995;75:484–7

15. Werfel T, Wedi B, Kleine-Tebbe J, et al How to manage a suspected pseudoallergic reaction to foods. Allergologie 2000;23:572–9
16. Asero R. Chronic unremitting urticaria: is the use of antihistamines above the licensed dose effective? A preliminary study of cetirizine at licensed and above-licensed doses. Clin Exp Dermatol. 2006;16:1–5
17. Simons FE, Sussman GL, Simons KJ. Effect of the H2-antagonist cimetidine on the pharmacokinetics and pharmacodynamics of the H1-antagonists hydroxyzine and cetirizine in patients with chronic urticaria. J Allergy Clin Immunol. 1995;95:685–93
18. Di Lorenzo G, Pacor ML, Mansueto P, et al Is there a role for antileukotrienes in urticaria? Clin Exp Dermatol. 2006;31:327–34
19. Grattan CE, O'Donnell BF, Francis DM, et al Randomized double-blind study of cyclosporin in chronic 'idiopathic' urticaria. Br J Dermatol. 2000;143:365–72
20. Dreskin SC, Andrews KY. The thyroid and urticaria. Curr Opin Allergy Clin Immunol. 2005;5:408–12
21. Shahar E, Bergman R, Guttman-Yassky E, et al Treatment of severe chronic idiopathic urticaria with oral mycophenolate mofetil in patients not responding to antihistamines and/or corticosteroids. Int J Dermatol. 2006;45:1224–7
22. Boyce JA. Successful treatment of cold-induced urticaria/anaphylaxis with anti-IgE. J Allergy Clin Immunol. 2006;117:1415–18

Standard Operating Procedures: A Practical Approach

7

M Metz and M Magerl

Core Messages

- Standard operating procedures (SOPs) offer guidance in which the diagnostic options seem to be countless. Furthermore, SOPs standardise diagnostic procedures. This is very important in key investigations when results have impact on the following treatment. Here, we present a selection of SOPs that are useful for the investigation of the underlying causes of chronic urticaria. These SOPs do not need to be adapted to specific requirements at different locations and can be used unmodified.
- The diagnosis of chronic urticaria is in general an unproblematic task: The presence of weals and/or angio-oedema, pruritus, and redness for more than 6 weeks will be recognised as chronic urticaria even by most untrained physicians.
- Far more difficult, however, is to objectively and reliably determine the urticaria subgroup the patient suffers from, and the time course and severity of the disease.
- The introduction of SOPs in the diagnosis of urticaria greatly improves the reliable, reproducible and observer-independent diagnosis of patients with chronic urticaria.
- The ICH GCP guidelines define SOP as “detailed, written instructions to achieve uniformity of the performance of a specific function”. It is of great importance to reach this “uniformity” in diagnosing urticaria subtypes and in assessing the severity of the disease, as treatment options may vary significantly depending on this information.
- In this chapter, we provide SOP used for the diagnosis of patients with chronic urticaria and describe the rationale for their use by hospital physicians as well as private practitioners.

M. Metz (✉)
Department of Dermatology and Allergy, Allergy-Centre-Charité, Charité-Universitätsmedizin Berlin, Charitéplatz 1, 10117 Berlin
e-mail: martin.metz@charite.de

T. Zuberbier et al. (eds.), *Urticaria and Angioedema*,
DOI: 10.1007/978-3-540-79048-8_7, © Springer Verlag Berlin Heidelberg 2010

7.1 Assessing Urticaria Activity Score

To be able to compare the results of clinical trials as well as of epidemiological investigations in patients with chronic urticaria, reliable symptom scores for assessing CU activity have to be used. Furthermore, an objective control of therapeutic and diagnostic measures, e.g. before and after performing a diet, before and after eradication of bacteria or before and after the start of a symptomatic treatment, also requires a standardised assessment of symptoms. The recent EAACI/EDF/GA²LEN/WAO guidelines recommend use of a straightforward and well-established symptom score, i.e. the urticaria activity score (UAS).

This simple scoring system is based on the assessment of key urticaria symptoms (weals and pruritus). Therefore, the questions addressed to the patients are:

How many weals have appeared during the last 24 h?	
Weals	Scoring
None	0
Mild (<20 weals/24 h)	1
Moderate (20–50 weals/24 h)	2
Intense (>50 weals/24 h or large confluent areas of weals)	3

How severe was the itch during the last 24 h?	
Itch	Scoring
None	0
Mild (present but not annoying or troublesome)	1
Moderate (troublesome but does not interfere with normal daily activity or sleep)	2
Intense (severe pruritus, which is sufficiently troublesome to interfere with normal daily activity or sleep)	3

Daily UAS is defined as the sum of the scoring values (score weals + score itch); the maximum daily UAS is 6. As urticaria symptoms frequently change in intensity during the course of a week, the overall disease activity is best measured by advising patients to document 24 h self-evaluation scores for 1 week [1]. The daily score sums are then summated to a weekly score, the maximum of which is 42.

7.2 Testing for Autoreactivity

In 1993, Hide et al. reported that the intracutaneous injection of serum, a procedure also known as autologous serum skin test (ASST), results in immediate hypersensitivity-type skin reactions in a subpopulation of CU patients [2]. This very simple and quick test can identify CU patients with circulating histamine-releasing factors, which has an important impact on the management of these patients. For example, it was found that ASST-positive patients exhibit a longer duration of disease and require markedly more antihistamines (about 2.5-fold) than ASST-negative patients, suggesting that ASST-positive CU patients may be less responsive to routine antihistamine therapy and may require a more intensified symptomatic treatment. Knowledge about the presence of histamine-releasing factors in the blood of CU patients thus provides the physician with valuable information affecting the further treatment of the CU patient. Furthermore, treatment options may vary considerably between ASST-positive and ASST-negative patients. For example, it has been reported that ASST-positive patients may benefit from treatment with autologous whole blood injections, while ASST-negative CU patients do not [3, 4].

To perform this test, the following material needs to be prepared:

- A timer, which can be set to at least half an hour
- A blood-drawing set with a serum vial, free from all coagulation-inducing substances
- Three single-use 1 ml syringes
- Several 0.8 mm needles to load the syringes
- Three 0.4 mm hypodermic needles for injection into the skin
- A centrifuge
- 0.9% Saline
- Histamine solution (0.1 mg/ml)

1. Venous blood should be collected into sterile glass tubes without accelerator or anticoagulant. Red-topped 7 ml BD Vacutainer® blood collection tubes (no additive) (Becton Dickinson, USA) are recommended. Blood should be allowed to clot at room temperature for 30 min before separation. Subsequently, the blood sample should be centrifuged at relative centrifugal force (RCF) of 450–500g (expressed in units of gravity) for 10 min. After the centrifuging, the sample tube is carefully removed and transported upright to the workstation.
2. The preparation of the injections takes place at a clean workstation. First, for the negative control injection, a 0.9% saline solution, drawn through a 0.8 mm cannula into a 1 ml syringe such as an insulin or tuberculin syringe and a 0.4 mm needle, suitable for intracutaneous injection, is attached. The protective covering remains on the needle. The syringe is marked with a permanent marker. The procedure for the positive control is the same. The histamine solution should be suitable for intracutaneous testing and should contain 0.1 mg/mL histamine.
3. Before the serum is drawn, the identity of the blood sample must be established without doubt. The slightest uncertainty means that the sample must be discarded. The drawing of the patient's serum takes place through a 0.8 mm cannula into a 1 ml syringe and a 0.4 mm needle, suitable for intracutaneous injection, is attached.
4. The volar forearm skin should be used after cleansing with antiseptic, avoiding the wrist and skin known to have had spontaneous weals in the previous 48 h (to avoid sites where mast cells may be refractory to further activation). The three testing areas (negative control, positive control, ASST) are labelled before the injections. The three test areas should be at least 3–5 cm apart. After the air has been expelled from the injection

system, the injection is strictly intracutaneous. 50 µl solution are injected, so that a lentil-sized welt forms. The injections should take place in rapid sequence.

5. Alternatively, the positive histamine control may be performed by skin prick testing (10 mg/ml).
6. The time of onset and initial appearance of a positive ASST response is similar to the response to intradermally injected histamine but the reaction persists for longer. Even though a 30 min reading for the ASST has become standard practice, a weal and flare response is usually apparent within 10 min and an additional 15 min reading has been performed in some centres. A positive ASST will often continue to enlarge with redness and a surrounding flare up to and beyond 30 min, whereas the saline control injection site will usually become flatter and remain pale. The reaction that is the diameter of the weal that has developed at the site of injection is measured with a transparent ruler. To be assessed as positive, the reaction to the serum must be 1.5 mm larger than the reaction to the negative control.

The re-injection of biological material to humans for diagnostic reasons should be performed under restrictively controlled conditions.

Only one person should be diagnosed at one site at one time-point.
All tubes/samples/syringes should be marked immediately and non-interchangeable
The slightest uncertainty means that the sample must be discarded!

7.3 Testing for Food Elicited Urticaria Diet

Adverse reactions to food are the cause of CU in a considerable number of patients. In general, both allergic and non-allergic reactions to food can be responsible for urticaria symptoms in these patients. However, while genuine IgE-dependent allergic reactions to food are known to play a role in acute urticaria (especially in young children), in some cases of exercise-induced urticaria, and in contact urticaria, it is largely negligible in chronic urticaria. Therefore, tests for food allergies (i.e. prick test, food antigen-specific IgE) are not useful in patients with chronic urticaria. Currently, only the conduction of a pseudoallergen-low diet can provide information on the presence of a CU due to food intolerance. This information is of great relevance for both physicians and patients as it can, on the one hand, lead to the development of an individual diet for those patients with food intolerance, which can result in the complete control of the CU symptoms, and on the other hand will give those patients who did not improve after the diet the certainty that they do not have to restrict their daily diet.

Before performing a pseudoallergen-low diet, the patients need to be informed thoroughly about:

- The meaning and importance of the diet
- The duration of at least 3 weeks

- That effects can be seen not until 10–14 days
- That each dietary "slip-up" can lessen the effectiveness
- That keeping a diary is obligatory
- That intake of antihistamines and glucocorticoids must be reduced to a minimum in order to judge the diet's outcome

After clarification of facts, the patient has to reorganise his complete alimentation for at least 3 weeks according to the list. During the diet, exclusively foods and drinks from the "allowed"-column must be ingested. All other foods – exemplified in the "forbidden" – column is strictly interdicted. If the patient is in doubt, the food should be banned.

	Allowed	Forbidden
Basic food	Additive-free bread, potatoes, rice, rice cakes, unprocessed cereals, flour (not self-raising!) durum wheat pasta (without egg)	All others (e. g. pasta with eggs, cake, biscuits, potato chips, crisps)
Fats	Butter, (cold pressed) plant oils	All others (e. g. margarine, mayonnaise)
Milk products	Fresh milk, cream without stabilisers, natural yoghurt, white cheese, fromage frais, a small amount of mild Gouda or butter cheese	All others
Food from animals	Fresh meat without seasoning	All others including eggs, sea-food, smoked meat
Vegetables	All except those listed as forbidden (e. g. lettuce, carrots, zucchini, cabbage, broccoli, asparagus)	Artichokes, peas, mushrooms, spinach, rhubarb, tomatoes and tomato products, olives, sweet peppers, spinach
Fruit	None	All including dried fruits or fruit juices
Herbs, spices	Salt, chives, onions	All others including garlic and herbs
Sweets	None, only sugar and honey	All including chewing gum
Beverages	Mineral water, coffee, black tea, green tea (without aroma)	All others including beer, wine, spirits and herbal teas

The following terms on an ingredient list indicate the presence of food additives: E100–E1518, colouring, preservative, gelling agents, thickening agents, moisturising agents, emulsifiers, flavour enhancers, antioxidants, separating agents, coatings, artificial sweeteners, baking agents, stabilisers, flour treatment agents, modified starches, foaming agents, artificial aroma.

7.4 Ins and Outs of the Food Labelling Rules

- According to the latest food labelling regulation (from 13 November 2004), sulphur dioxide and sulphites must be listed on food packaging if the concentration is higher than 10 mg/kg or l. This means sulphur dioxide and sulphites may be present in food, but undeclared. Also, be careful with foods that are not pre-packaged.

- The following food products may contain additives that are not listed on the label:
  - Unpacked processed food products (e.g. bread, cake, cookies, sausage, salads)
  - Potato products (e.g. chips or croquettes) from take-away shops
  - Alcoholic drinks
  - Chocolates or pralines.
  - You can ask about additives at the meat or cheese counter, there must be a folder where additives are listed.
  - *Warning*: No labelling is required for additives composed of different ingredients, when the resulting mixture does not affect the texture or flavour of the food (exceptions are sulphur dioxide and sulphites).

7.5 Use of Diary Cards

The exact documentation of the daily symptoms in combination with the record of the intake of drugs, unusual food, physical or emotional stress or other conspicuous situations can lead to the identification of factors that induce or exacerbate urticaria in the individual patient. The keeping of a diary can be especially helpful for patients with varying severity of symptoms or patients with episodic attacks of urticaria and for patients who perform a diagnostic diet.

Depending on the patients' symptoms, the diary can be kept in the form of a monthly calendar with daily record of symptoms for multiple months or as an episode protocol intended for the daily record of symptoms for days to weeks.

1. Month (Fig. 7.1)
2. Episode protocol (Fig. 7.2)

7.6 Questionnaire

The careful and precise documentation of the medical history of a patient with chronic urticaria is of prime importance. The evaluation of an accurately performed medical history can lead to the identification of an underlying cause of the urticaria, will give important hints on treatment possibilities and will help to plan the next diagnostic steps. Therefore, standardized questionnaires for the assessment of the medical history are recommended:

Urticaria-Calendar

This calendar can help you to monitor the course of your urticaria and to find factors/triggers that may induce or aggravate your symptoms. Please indicate once a day 1) how many wheals occured, 2) how itchy your skin was, 3) whether you had additional symptoms (and if so, how strong they were) and 4) whether (and when) you administered your anti-histaminic medication.

The prescribed anti-histamine is*:_ ________________________ ___

Day	Wheals				Itch				Other Symptoms				Anti-histamines*				Triggers
	none	<20	20-50	>50	none	lightly	medium	strong	none	low	strong	maximum	morning	noon	afternoon	at night	For example: - Stress - Exercise - Food
1																	
2																	
3																	
4																	
5																	
6																	
7																	
8																	
9																	
10																	
11																	
12																	
13																	
14																	
15																	
16																	
17																	
18																	
19																	
20																	
21																	
22																	
23																	
24																	
25																	
26																	
27																	
28																	
29																	
30																	
31																	

Fig. 7.1 Monthly urticaria calender (ECARF, used with permission)

	How many wheals/ erythem as have appeared during the last 24 hours?	What size did most of these wheals / erythem as have during the last 24 hours?	For how many hours did you have wheals / erythem as during the last 24 hours?	For how many hours did the longest-lasting wheals / erythem as Keep up during the last 24 hours?	Where there large confluent areas of wheals during thelast 24 hours?
Wheals yes → / ☐ no	☐ <20 ☐ 20-50 ☐ >50	☐ <1 cm ☐ 1-5 cm ☐ >5 cm	☐ <3 hours ☐ 3-12 hours ☐ >12 hours	☐ <3 hours ☐ 3-24 hours ☐ >24 hours	☐ yes ☐ no
Erythema yes → / ☐ no	☐ <20 ☐ 20-50 ☐ >50	☐ <1 cm ☐ 1-5 cm ☐ >5 cm	☐ <3 hours ☐ 3-12 hours ☐ >12 hours	☐ <3 hours ☐ 3-24 hours ☐ >24 hours	

	Please choose the category that best describes your angioedema(s) during the last 24 hours?	How severe were the complaints caused by edema during the last 24 hours?
Angioedema yes → / ☐ no	☐ small / mild ☐ moderate ☐ large / severe	☐ mild ☐ moderate ☐ severe

	How many hours did you experience itch during the last 24 hours?	How severe was the itch during the last 24 hours?
Itch / Pruritus yes → / ☐ no	☐ <3 hours ☐ 3-12 hours ☐ >12 hours	☐ mild ☐ moderate ☐ severe

Please rate the severity of your urticaria complaints:

☐ no complaints ☐ mild complaints ☐ moderate complaints ☐ severe complaints

Intake of antihistamines due to unbearable itch:

drug (dose in mg) ____________________ intake (e.g. 1-0-1-0) (morning noon evening night) ____________________

____________________ ____________________

Intake of other drugs:

drug (dose in mg) ____________________ intake (e.g. 1-0-1-0) ____________________

Have you taken your prescribed drugs as usual?

☐ yes ☐ no, because ____________________

Please note possible triggers of your urticaria symptoms:

____

____

____

____

____

____

____

____

____

____

____

Fig. 7.2 Urticaria episode protocol (ECARF, used with permission)

Medical History Questionnaire

To find out what could be responsible for your urticaria, it is necessary that your doctor has as much information on the course of your urticaria as possible. This is why we ask you to fill out this questionnaire. It is very important to read the questions carefully.

1. Since when do you have your urticaria?
2. Do you think that there was a specific reason or trigger for your urticaria when it started? What do you make responsible for the onset of your urticaria?
3. Please name the average size, duration and location of your weals or of your swellings? How strong is your itchiness usually?
4. When and how do weals or swellings appear? (What days of the week, time of day, season?)
5. Are there any other symptoms that go together with your weals or swellings such as breathlessness, headaches or gastrointestinal problems?
6. Do you presently have other medical problems? If yes: What kind of medical problems?
7. Does or did anybody in your family also have urticaria?
8. Do you suffer any other allergies?
9. What do you think could be triggering or worsening your urticaria attacks (for example: stress, physical exercise, food, medication, sun, pressure on the skin, cold or hot temperatures)?
10. Do you currently use any medication? If yes, what kind, which dosage, since when?
11. What kind of medication do you use when you have a headache and how does it help?
12. What kind of medication do you take for your urticaria and how does it help?
13. What do you do professionally? Do you think that your job has something to do with your urticaria?
14. What kind of hobbies do you have? Could this have anything to do with your urticaria?
15. Does your urticaria affect your quality of life? If so, how and how much?

Please feel free to provide additional information that you think your doctor may find helpful for understanding you and your urticaria.

7.7 Prick Test

Allergies are often thought by patients to be a frequent underlying cause of chronic urticaria. Although this is not the case, a standardised prick test should be performed on patients with chronic urticaria to definitely rule out an allergic context and, in those patients with sensitisations to allergens, to assess co-morbidity of urticaria and allergies. Skin prick testing is the standard method for diagnosing allergic sensitisation and should be performed according to standard protocols to facilitate comparisons of sensitisations throughout different clinical centres and countries.

GA²LEN Protocol for Pan-European Skin prick test

The following points have to be observed:

1. A standard list of allergens will be used. Each subject will be skin tested using the following panel of allergens:

(1) Histamine
(2) Negative control
(3) Hazel
(4) Alder
(5) Birch
(6) Plane
(7) Cypress
(8) Grass mix
(9) Olive
(10) Artemisia
(11) Ambrosia
(12) Alternaria
(13) Cladosporium
(14) Aspergillus
(15) Parietaria
(16) Cat
(17) Dog
(18) Dermatophagoides pteronyssinus
(19) Dermatophagoides farinae
(20) Blatella

Only if medical history reveals a well-founded suspicion of another allergic background of the urticaria, the panel should be expanded by the corresponding allergens.

Positive control: histamine 1:100
Negative control: diluent

2. Skin test solutions must be stored at +2 to +8°C when not in use.
3. Place a clean test grid on volar surface of the forearm and fix with tape. Mark the orientation of the grid on the subject's arm.
4. Place a small drop of each skin testing solution in the centre of each grid square. Apply the skin test allergens in the same order during each test.
5. Press the lancet through the drop against the skin for at least 1 s. Always apply the same pressure. The skin should not be broken to the extent that blood is drawn.
6. Use a new lancet for each allergen.
7. Remove the skin test grid. Blot any excess solution with a tissue taking care not to cross-contaminate the tests.
8. Set the timer alarm and read the results after 15 min.
9. Measure the largest and the perpendicular diameter of the weal of each of the allergens. Calculate the value: Largest + perpendicular diameter/2 (for example $(5 + 3)/2 = 4$). Document the patient's data (Fig. 7.3).
10. Assess the relevance of each of the positively tested allergens (0 = no relevance; 1 = relevant; 2 = former relevance; 3 = unknown).

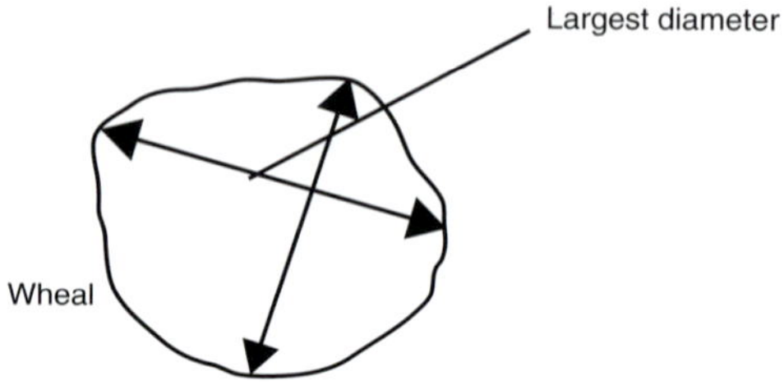

Fig. 7.3 Assessment of prick test (ECARF, used with permission)

7.8
Take Home Pearls

- The Urticaria Activity Score (UAS) is a useful instrument to assess the severity of chronic urticaria. Therapeutic effects can be measured sensitively.
- Patients with autoreactive urticaria are readily identified by the autologous serum skin test, in which they exhibit inflammatory reactions to their serum after intracutaneous injection. This test is simple and quick.
- Patients with food elicited urticaria can be helped by a diet low in pseudoallergens. Almost 50% of the patients are convinced that food plays a role in urticaria, in 30% this suspicion is confirmed by diet.
- Diary: The easiest way to find triggers and underlying causes. Helps to assess severity and to detect patterns of skin rashing. Very helpful to perform purposeful investigations.
- Medical History: Plays a key role in all urticaria patients, but may be very complex in many patients. Therefore, a standardised questionnaire (to be filled before the clinic) helps one to answer important questions quickly.
- Skin prick test: Allergic urticaria is not very common. However, if the suspicion has aroused, prick test helps to rule out (or to confirm) allergic reactions.

References

1. Młynek A et al How to assess disease activity in patients with chronic urticaria? Allergy 2008;63(6):777–80
2. Hide M, Francis DM, Grattan CE, Hakimi J, Kochan JP, Greaves MW Autoantibodies against the high-affinity IgE receptor as a cause of histamine release in chronic urticaria. N Engl J Med. 1993 Jun 3;328(22):1599–604
3. Staubach P, Onnen K, Vonend A, Metz M, Siebenhaar F, Tschentscher I, Opper B, Magerl M, Lüdtke R, Kromminga A, Maurer M Autologous whole blood injections to patients with chronic urticaria and a positive autologous serum skin test: a placebo-controlled trial. Dermatology. 2006;212(2):150–9
4. Konstantinou GN, Asero R, Maurer M, Sabroe RA, Schmid-Grendelmeier P, Grattan CE The following protocol is recommended by an EAACI/GA2LEN taskforce Allergy. 2009 Sep; 64(9):1256–68

Appendix

Recommended Treatment Algorithm for Chronic Urticaria which is part of the New 2009 International Guideline on Urticaria

The guideline is the result of a consensus conference and discussions between an expert panel and more than 200 practicing specialists in the field. The stepwise approach in the algorithm is based on the evidence level available for the different drug interventions but is also taking into consideration the safety profile and the costs. The following considerations have been made for the different levels:

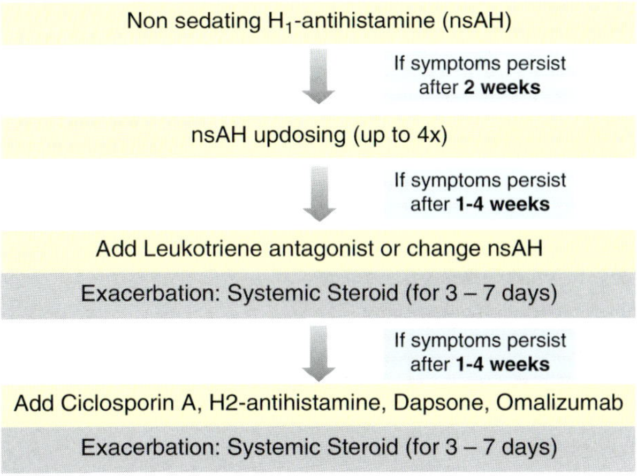

Comments on procedure on algorithm for chronic urticaria

First Level: High quality evidence

- Low cost (worldwide availability also in developing countries mostly cheaper than old sedating antihistamines)
- Very good safety profile
- Very good evidence for efficacy

T. Zuberbier et al. (eds.), *Urticaria and Angioedema*,
DOI: 10.1007/978-3-540-79048-8_Appendix, © Springer Verlag Berlin Heidelberg 2010

Second level: low-quality evidence

- Low cost
- Good safety profile
- Good evidence for efficacy

Third level: very-low-quality evidence

- Low to medium–low cost
- Good safety profile
- Insufficient or no evidence for efficacy in high-quality RCT

Fourth level:

- Ciclosporin A:
  - Medium to high cost
  - Moderate safety profile
  - Moderate level of evidence for efficacy
- H2-Antihistamine:
  - Low cost
  - Good safety profile
  - Very low level of evidence for efficacy
- Dapsone:
  - Low cost
  - Medium level of side effects
  - Low level of evidence for efficacy
- Anti-IgE:
  - High cost
  - Good safety profile
  - Low level evidence for good efficacy

Index